Jacqueline Garrick, CSW, ACSW, BCETS
Mary Beth Williams, PhD, LCSW, CTS
Editors

Trauma Treatment Techniques: Innovative Trends

Trauma Treatment Techniques: Innovative Trends has been co-published simultaneously as *Journal of Aggression, Maltreatment & Trauma*, Volume 12, Numbers 1/2, 2006.

Pre-publication
REVIEWS,
COMMENTARIES,
EVALUATIONS . . .

"This book OFFERS A BROAD VIEW OF INNOVATIONS IN THE FIELD AND A VALUABLE GLIMPSE OF WHAT LIES JUST BEYOND THE HORIZON. Two established leaders in the practice of psychological trauma therapy provide a survey of approaches that are 'on the edge.' The inclusiveness of this book is its great virtue. Researchers and clinicians may differ among themselves and between groups about what constitutes scientific theory or appropriate clinical practice but the field needs an articulate compendium of new therapeutic initiatives and Garrick and Williams have delivered."

Harold Kudler, MD
Associate Clinical Professor
Department of Psychiatry
and Behavioral Services
Duke University

More Pre-publication
REVIEWS, COMMENTARIES, EVALUATIONS . . .

"THIS IS AN OUTSTANDING BOOK that will inform the novice as well as the seasoned clinician about innovative treatments for traumatic stress. . . . Provides the reader with an incredibly broad perspective on available treatments. The book features many innovative and state-of-the-art topics for treatment of PTSD, ASD, and dissociative disorders. Not only does it describe many of these innovative theories, it also provides a practical, 'how-to' approach for administration of these therapeutic techniques. The book will inform students and clinicians about alternative approaches for the successful resolution of PTSD. In particular, the chapter by Ronald T. Murphy and Craig S. Rosen provides the reader with important information about preparing the trauma survivor to identify problem behaviors and about building a rationale for the resolution of symptoms. In addition, Mary Beth Williams' chapter on responding to school violence provides practical guidance and should be read by any therapist or grief counselor who participates in school or classroom debriefing."

Greg Leskin, PhD
National Center for PTSD,
VA Palo Alto Healthcare System

"This collection SIGNIFICANTLY BROADENS THE UNDERSTANDING OF INNOVATIVE TECHNIQUES FOR THE TREATMENT OF PTSD AND ASSOCIATED CONDITIONS. It contains clear descriptions of new treatments for PTSD which include residential treatment; thought field therapy; acute stress debriefing in schools; emotional freedom techniques, and virtual reality therapy for war veterans. This book should be read by all who seek new knowledge and creative applications of nontraditional approaches to working with trauma victims. It foreshadows the next wave in posttraumatic therapies and clinical innovations that move beyond the limitations of conventional treatment approaches."

John P. Wilson
Fulbright Scholar and Professor of Psychology, Cleveland State University; Co-Founder and Past President, International Society for Traumatic Stress Studies; Co-Director, International Institute on Psychotraumatology

Shaken Baby Syndrome (SBS). Offers expert information and advice on every aspect of prevention, diagnosis, treatment, and follow-up.

Trauma and Cognitive Science: A Meeting of Minds, Science, and Human Experience, edited by Jennifer J. Freyd, PhD, and Anne P. DePrince, MS (Vol. 4, No. 2 [#8] 2001). *"A fine collection of scholarly works that address key questions about memory for childhood and adult traumas from a variety of disciplines and empirical approaches. A must-read volume for anyone wishing to understand traumatic memory." (Kathryn Quina, PhD, Professor of Psychology & Women's Studies, University of Rhode Island)*

Program Evaluation and Family Violence Research, edited by Sally K. Ward, PhD, and David Finkelhor, PhD (Vol. 4, No. 1 [#7], 2000). *"Offers wise advice to evaluators and others interested in understanding the impact of their work. I learned a lot from reading this book." (Jeffrey L. Edleson, PhD, Professor, University of Minnesota, St. Paul)*

Sexual Abuse Litigation: A Practical Resource for Attorneys, Clinicians, and Advocates, edited by Rebecca Rix, MALS (Vol. 3, No. 2 [#6], 2000). *"An interesting and well developed treatment of the complex subject of child sexual abuse trauma. The merger of the legal, psychological, scientific and historical expertise of the authors provides a unique, in-depth analysis of delayed discovery in CSA litigation. This book, including the extremely useful appendices, is a must for the attorney or expert witness who is involved in the representation of survivors of sexual abuse." (Leonard Karp, JD, and Cheryl L. Karp, PhD, co-authors, Domestic Torts: Family Violence, Conflict and Sexual Abuse)*

Children Exposed to Domestic Violence: Current Issues in Research, Intervention, Prevention, and Policy Development, edited by Robert A. Geffner, PhD, Peter G. Jaffe, PhD, and Marlies Sudermann, PhD (Vol. 3, No. 1 [#5], 2000). *"A welcome addition to the resource library of every professional whose career encompasses issues of children's mental health, well-being, and best interest . . . I strongly recommend this helpful and stimulating text." (The Honorable Justice Grant A. Campbell, Justice of the Ontario Superior Court of Justice, Family Court, London, Canada)*

Maltreatment in Early Childhood: Tools for Research-Based Intervention, edited by Kathleen Coulborn Faller, PhD (Vol. 2, No. 2 [#4], 1999). *"This important book takes an international and cross-cultural look at child abuse and maltreatment. Discussing the history of abuse in the United States, exploring psychological trauma, and containing interviews with sexual abuse victims,* Maltreatment in Early Childhood *provides counselors and mental health practitioners with research that may help prevent child abuse or reveal the mistreatment some children endure."*

Multiple Victimization of Children: Conceptual, Developmental, Research, and Treatment Issues, edited by B. B. Robbie Rossman, PhD, and Mindy S. Rosenberg, PhD (Vol. 2, No. 1 [#3], 1998). *"This book takes on a large challenge and meets it with stunning success. It fills a glaring gap in the literature . . . " (Edward P. Mulvey, PhD, Associate Professor of Child Psychiatry, Western Psychiatric Institute and Clinic, University of Pittsburgh School of Medicine)*

Violence Issues for Health Care Educators and Providers, edited by L. Kevin Hamberger, PhD, Sandra K. Burge, PhD, Antonnette V. Graham, PhD, and Anthony J. Costa, MD (Vol. 1, No. 2 [#2], 1997). *"A superb book that contains invaluable hands-on advice for medical educators and health care professionals alike . . . " (Richard L. Holloways, PhD, Professor and Vice Chair, Department of Family and Community Medicine, and Associate Dean for Student Affairs, Medical College of Wisconsin)*

Violence and Sexual Abuse at Home: Current Issues in Spousal Battering and Child Maltreatment, edited by Robert Geffner, PhD, Susan B. Sorenson, PhD, and Paula K. Lundberg-Love, PhD (Vol. 1, No. 1 [#1], 1997). *"The Editors have distilled the important questions at the cutting edge of the field of violence studies, and have brought rigor, balance and moral fortitude to the search for answers." (Virginia Goldner, PhD, Co-Director, Gender and Violence Project, Senior Faculty, Ackerman Institute for Family Therapy)*

Trauma Treatment Techniques:
Innovative Trends

Jacqueline Garrick, CSW, ACSW, BCETS
Mary Beth Williams, PhD, LCSW, CTS
Editors

Trauma Treatment Techniques: Innovative Trends has been co-published simultaneously as *Journal of Aggression, Maltreatment & Trauma*, Volume 12, Numbers 1/2, 2006.

HMTP

The Haworth Maltreatment & Trauma Press®
An Imprint of The Haworth Press, Inc.

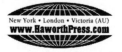

New York • London • Victoria (AU)
www.HaworthPress.com

Published by

The Haworth Maltreatment & Trauma Press, 10 Alice Street, Binghamton, NY 13904-1580 USA

The Haworth Maltreatment & Trauma Press is an imprint of The Haworth Press, Inc., 10 Alice Street, Binghamton, NY 13904-1580 USA.

Trauma Treatment Techniques: Innovative Trends has been co-published simultaneously as *Journal of Aggression, Maltreatment & Trauma*, Volume 12, Numbers 1/2 2006.

The development, preparation, and publication of this work has been undertaken with great care. However, the publisher, employees, editors, and agents of The Haworth Press and all imprints of The Haworth Press, Inc., including The Haworth Medical Press® and The Pharmaceutical Products Press®, are not responsible for any errors contained herein or for consequences that may ensue from use of materials or information contained in this work. Opinions expressed by the author(s) are not necessarily those of The Haworth Press, Inc. With regard to case studies, identities and circumstances of individual discussed herein have been changed to protect confidentiality. Any resemblance to actual persons, living or dead, is entirely coincidental.

Cover design by Lora Wiggins

Library of Congress Cataloging-in-Publication Data

Trauma treatment techniques : innovative trends/ Jacqueline Garrick, Mary Beth Williams, editors.
     p. cm.
    "Co-published simultaneously as Journal of aggression, maltreatment & trauma, volume 12, numbers 1/2 2006."
    Includes bibliographical references and index.
    ISBN-13: 978-0-7890-2843-3 (hc. : alk.paper)
    ISBN-10: 0-7890-2843-3 (hc. : alk.paper)
    ISBN-13: 978-0-7890-2844-0 (pbk. : alk.paper)
    ISBN-10: 0-7890-2844-1 (pbk. : alk.paper)
    1. Post-traumatic stress disorder–Treatment. 2. Psychic trauma–Treatment. I. Garrick, Jacqueline, CSW. II. Williams, Mary Beth.
  RC552. P67T75532006
  616.85′2106–dc22
                                         2006027129

Indexing, Abstracting & Website/Internet Coverage

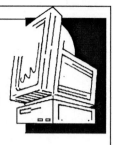

This section provides you with a list of major indexing & abstracting services and other tools for bibliographic access. That is to say, each service began covering this periodical during the year noted in the right column. Most Websites which are listed below have indicated that they will either post, disseminate, compile, archive, cite or alert their own Website users with research-based content from this work. (This list is as current as the copyright date of this publication.)

Abstracting, Website/Indexing Coverage . . . . Year When Coverage Began

- *Business Source Corporate: coverage of nearly 3,350 quality magazines and journals; designed to meet the diverse infromation needs of corporations; EBSCO Publishing <http://www.epnet.com/corporate/bsource.asp>* **2002**

- *Cambridge Scientific Abstracts is a leading publisher of scientific information in print journals, online databases, CD-ROM and via the Internet <http://www.csa.com>* **1997**

- *Caredata: the database supporting social care management and practice <http://www.elsc.org.uk/caredata/caredata.htm>* **1998**

- *Child Development Abstracts & Bibliography (in print and online) <http://www.ukans.edu>* **1997**

- *CINAHL (Cumulative Index to Nursing & Allied Health Literature), in print, EBSCO, and SilverPlatter, Data-Star, and PaperChase. (Support materials include Subject Heading List, Database Search Guide, and instructional video) <http://www.cinahl.com>* **2000**

- *Criminal Justice Abstracts.* **1997**

- *e-psyche, LLC <http://www.e-psyche.net>* **2001**

- *EBSCOhost Electronic Journals Service (EJS) <http://ejournals.ebsco.com>* **2002**

(continued)

(continued)

Special Bibliographic Notes related to special journal issues (separates) and indexing/abstracting:

- indexing/abstracting services in this list will also cover material in any "separate" that is co-published simultaneously with Haworth's special thematic journal issue or DocuSerial. Indexing/abstracting usually covers material at the article/chapter level.
- monographic co-editions are intended for either non-subscribers or libraries which intend to purchase a second copy for their circulating collections.
- monographic co-editions are reported to all jobbers/wholesalers/approval plans. The source journal is listed as the "series" to assist the prevention of duplicate purchasing in the same manner utilized for books-in-series.
- to facilitate user/access services all indexing/abstracting services are encouraged to utilize the co-indexing entry note indicated at the bottom of the first page of each article/chapter/contribution.
- this is intended to assist a library user of any reference tool (whether print, electronic, online, or CD-ROM) to locate the monographic version if the library has purchased this version but not a subscription to the source journal.
- individual articles/chapters in any Haworth publication are also available through the Haworth Document Delivery Service (HDDS).

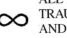

ABOUT THE EDITORS

Jacqueline Garrick, CSW, ACSW, BCETS, has her own consulting business, the FARgroup, in Silver Spring, Maryland and is primarily providing policy analysis, strategic planning, fundraising, program development and evaluation support to nonprofit, private and government entities. She is a former Army Social Work Officer and was the Deputy Director for Health Care at The American Legion. She has lectured on trauma throughout the United States and Europe.

Mary Beth Williams, PhD, LCSW, CTS, is in private practice in Warrenton, Virginia. A former school social worker, she now devotes her time to private practice, to teaching both nationally and internationally, to consulting with various organizations including the Crisis Team of the EPA, and to her newly adopted daughters from Kazakhstan.

Trauma Treatment Techniques: Innovative Trends

CONTENTS

ABOUT THE CONTRIBUTORS

Renato D. Alarcon, MD, MPH, is currently Professor of Psychiatry at Mayo Medical School, Director of the Teaching Unit at Mayo Medical Center, and Medical Director of the Mayo Psychiatry and Psychology Treatment Center. A native of Peru, he completed his residency at Johns Hopkins, and has worked at the University of Alabama at Birmingham and at Emory University prior to his current position. He is the author of more than 160 articles, author or editor of twelve books and more than fifty book chapters. His areas of clinical and academic interest are mood and personality disorders, PTSD, and cultural psychiatry.

Barbara Ann Baker, MA-AT, is an art therapist at Florida Hospital Center for Behavior Health, a crisis center for adolescents and adults in Orlando, Florida. Her background includes working with multicultural populations, refugees, and the mentally ill at Chicago Health Outreach in Chicago. Ms. Baker has given presentations, workshops, and been a consultant. She received her BA at the University of Central Florida and her MA-AT at the University of Illinois at Chicago. Ms. Baker has been recognized as an artist who has exhibited, won many awards, and has art in permanent collections. She has two adult sons and lives in Winter Park, Florida.

Dr. James Ball is Vice President of Autism Services for YCS, a not-for-profit social services agency located in New Jersey. He operates six private schools, working with over 200 students and their families affected with autism spectrum disorders. He has his doctorate from Nova Southeastern University and has been working in the field of autism for over 20 years. He has lectured nationally and internationally on topics related to autism spectrum disorders and has published in the areas of integrated preschool, accountability, and teaching social skills.

Robert Bray, PhD, LCSW, is a certified trauma specialist, President of the Association for Thought Field Therapy, President of the Association of Traumatic Stress Specialists, an approved International Critical Incident Stress Foundation trainer, faculty at San Diego State University School of Social Work, and has been in private practice since 1986 specializing in traumatic stress recovery.

Dr. Walter Busuttil, MB, ChB, MPhil, MRCGP, MRCPsych, is a consultant psychiatrist and Director of the Trauma Service at The Priory, Ticehurst House Hospital, East Sussex, England. He is Honorary Senior Lecturer in Psychiatry to the Kent Institute of Medicine and Health Sciences of the University of Kent at Canterbury. He is a military psychiatrist by background, having served for sixteen years in Royal Air Force where he played a key role in the setting up novel PTSD rehabilitation programs after the 1991 Gulf War. He also formed part of the team that helped to rehabilitate the British hostages released from Beirut in 1991and the British Gulf War POWs. Since joining the Trauma Service at Ticehurst in 1997, he has continued to develop group rehabilitation programs for traumatic stress victims and maintained his interest in group rehabilitation programs, as well as the rehabilitation of family members of those involved in catastrophic stress. He has published numerous scientific papers in posttraumatic stress and has contributed to leading textbooks. He lectures widely in these fields in the United Kingdom and internationally.

Garry A. Flint, PhD, is a registered psychologist in private practice in Vernon, British Columbia, Canada. He has 28 years of experience as a therapist and has had training in several energy psychology approaches. He is currently engaged in the theoretical analysis of energy psychology methods. He has developed a treatment approach that facilitates working with dissociative patients. A description of this approach can be found on *http://www.process-healing.com*

Dan Gillette received his BA from the Lesley College Graduate School and his EdM from the Harvard University Graduate School of Education. He is the chair of the Innovative Technology for Autism Committee at Cure Autism Now. Mr. Gillette consults in education, product design and disability, and is an academic specialist at the Institute of Urban and Regional Development (IURD) at UC Berkeley.

Frank Gerbode, MD, obtained his BA with honors in Philosophy from Stanford in 1962, his MD from Yale Medical School in 1968, and completed his psychiatric training at Stanford in 1972. He founded the Institute for Research in Metapsychology (now Applied Metapsychology

International–AMI) in 1986. Since that time, with his colleagues, he has been pursuing his interest in finding helping methods that are easy to learn and to apply. TIR is one of those methods.

Chrys J. Harris, PhD, is a licensed marriage and family therapist, a licensed professional counselor, a diplomate of the American Board of Forensic Examiners, a diplomate of the American Board of Psychological Specialties (Trauma/PTSD), a member of the American Academy of Experts in Traumatic Stress, and a certified trauma specialist. He is Clinical Director of the Family Therapy and Trauma Center in Greer, South Carolina. Dr. Harris maintains a private practice specializing in marriage and family therapy; he is also a forensic consultant in emotional trauma.

Willem Lammers, TSTA, CTS, is a social and clinical psychologist, and a licensed psychotherapist, with over 20 years of experience in the field. He is a consultant to organizations. He is a certified teaching and supervising transactional analyst and an ATSS certified trauma specialist. He is currently Director of IAS, the Institute for the Application of the Social Sciences in Maienfeld, Switzerland. After training in the USA he has been working with meridian-based psychotherapies since 1996 and developed several new techniques and applications. He is the ACEP representative for mainland Europe and teaches in many different countries.

Deborah G. Mitnick, MSW, LCSW-C, is a psychotherapist in private practice who specializes in treatments aimed at rapid emotional healing. She also provides personal performance coaching and trauma relief services. She is a supervisor in Critical Incident Stress Debriefing at Sheppard Pratt Psychiatric Hospital in Baltimore, Maryland, USA, and is a national consultant to crisis management companies. Her Web page is *http://www.trauma-tir.com*

Ronald Murphy, PhD, is currently Assistant Professor in the Department of Psychology at Dillard University in New Orleans. Dr. Murphy's research interests include the effectiveness of motivation enhancement approaches for combat-related PTSD, predictors of PTSD treatment outcome, and racism-related stress. His recent publications include articles on psychological assessment, motivation to change among veterans in PTSD treatment, patient response to the PTSD ME

Group, and predictors of stress symptoms among college students after the September 11 terror attacks.

Dr. Robert Naseef is a psychologist in independent practice in Philadelphia and a consultant to numerous schools and human service organizations. Dr. Naseef's specialty is working with families of children with special health care needs. He serves on the Board of Directors of the Center for Autistic Children and is author of *Special Children, Challenged Parents: The Struggles and Rewards of Parenting a Child With a Disability*, and is the parent of an adult child with autism.

Ron Oberleitner is President of e-Merge Medical Technologies, Technology Advisor to nonprofit Princeton Autism Technology (Princeton, NJ), and General Manager of TalkAutism Communication Service. With over 15 years leading Product Development and Marketing in the medical device industry, Mr. Oberleitner has developed many new technologies and services for various medical populations. He is the father of an eleven-year-old son with autism.

Dr. Stacey Pollack is the director of the PTSD program at the Washington DC VA Medical Center. She is also the director of the DC VA Medical Center's mental health disaster response team. Dr. Pollack received her BA from the University of Maryland-College Park, and her MS and PhD from the University of Georgia. At present, Dr. Pollack is involved in research utilizing exposure therapy to treat combat veterans with PTSD.

David J. Ready, PhD, is the psychologist for the Posttraumatic Stress Disorder Clinical Team of the Atlanta VA Medical Center and is Assistant Professor, Clinical Track, in the Department of Psychiatry and Behavioral Sciences, Emory School of Medicine. Dr. Ready received a grant from the Emory University Research Committee to conduct the second open VRE trial. Dr. Ready has 18 years of VA experience and is interested in developing more effective treatment models for veterans suffering from PTSD.

Craig Rosen, PhD, is a clinical psychologist and health services researcher specializing in recovery from psychological trauma. Dr. Rosen is Assistant Professor of Psychiatry and Behavioral Sciences at the Stanford University School of Medicine, and a health science specialist at the Menlo Park division of the Department of Veterans Affairs (VA) National Center for Posttraumatic Stress Disorder. Dr. Rosen is also affiliated with the VA Sierra-Pacific Mental Illness Research, Education, and Clinical Center, the Stanford/VA Center for Health Care Evaluation, and Stanford/VA Alzheimer's Research Center of California. Dr. Rosen's research interests include patient readiness for change, quality of care for veterans with PTSD, crisis counseling services for survivors of disasters and terrorism, comorbid substance use and traumatic stress, and translation of science into clinical practice.

Barbara Olasov Rothbaum, PhD, received her doctorate in clinical psychology in 1986 and is currently a tenured associate professor in psychiatry at the Emory School of Medicine in the Department of Psychiatry and Behavioral Sciences, and Director of the Trauma and Anxiety Recovery Program at Emory. Dr. Rothbaum specializes in research on the treatment of individuals with anxiety disorders, particularly focusing on Posttraumatic Stress Disorder (PTSD). She has won both state and national awards for her research, is an invited speaker internationally, authors scientific papers and chapters, has published two books on the treatment of PTSD, and received the Diplomate in Behavioral Psychology from the American Board of Professional Psychology. She is on the Board of Directors of the International Society of Traumatic Stress Studies (ISTSS), is President of ISTSS, and is Associate Editor of *The Journal of Traumatic Stress*. Dr. Rothbaum is also a pioneer in the application of virtual reality to the treatment of psychological disorders.

B. Hudnall Stamm, PhD, educated in psychology and statistics at Appalachian State University (BS, MA) and University of Wyoming (PhD), is a research professor, Director of Telehealth, and Deputy Director of the Idaho State University Institute of Rural Health. Working primarily with rural underserved peoples, Stamm's efforts focus on health policy, cultural trauma, and work-related traumatic stress where telehealth figures prominently. The author over one hundred professional documents, her books include *Measurement of Stress, Trauma and Adaptation* (1995, Sidran Press), *Cultural Issues and the Treatment of Trauma and Loss* (with Nader & Dubrow, 1999, Brunner/Mazel), *Secondary Traumatic Stress* (1995/1999, Sidran Press), and *Rural Behavioral Healthcare* (2003, APA Books).

Introduction

Jacqueline Garrick

SUMMARY. The introduction provides an overview of this volume. *Trauma Treatment Techniques: Innovative Trends* was developed based on the recognition that there are various approaches to mitigating the symptoms of traumatic stress. The introduction describes several techniques that use non-traditional or augment "talk therapy." The techniques are described by the experts in their particular practice arena. *[Article copies available for a fee from The Haworth Document Delivery Service: 1-800-HAWORTH. E-mail address: <docdelivery@haworthpress.com> Website: <http://www.Haworth Press. com> © 2006 by The Haworth Press, Inc. All rights reserved.]*

KEYWORDS. Trauma treatment, techniques, therapy

Throughout the course of human events, individuals have had to confront terrible events and stressful hardships. Anthropologists have studied the etchings of prehistoric man and Egyptian Hieroglyphics to understand how these cultures survived or perished in times of flood, famine, fighting, or other disasters. Why they left behind these markings is speculative, but this need to "tell a story" is obvious. As man evolved, the need to understand self in context of the environment emerged, as in the writings of Plato and Homer. As

Address correspondence to Jacqueline Garrick, CSW, ACSW, BCETS, 2 Narrows Court, SilverSpring, MD 20906 (E-mail: cptjax@aol.com).

[Haworth co-indexing entry note]: "Introduction." Garrick, Jacqueline. Co-published simultaneously in *Journal of Aggression, Maltreatment & Trauma* (The Haworth Maltreatment & Trauma Press, an imprint of The Haworth Press, Inc.) Vol. 12, No. 1/2, 2006, pp. 1-6; and: *Trauma Treatment Techniques: Innovative Trends* (ed: Jacqueline Garrick, and Mary Beth Williams) The Haworth Maltreatment & Trauma Press, an imprint of The Haworth Press, Inc., 2006, pp. 1-6. Single or multiple copies of this article are available for a fee from The Haworth Document Delivery Service [1-800-HAWORTH, 9:00 a.m. - 5:00 p.m. (EST). E-mail address: docdelivery@haworthpress.com].

doi:10.1300/J146v12n01_01

the need to understand life's meaning and purpose emerged throughout various cultures, so did the need for religion, education, science and psychology. The need to "tell a story" is the catalyst for how to "listen to a story," which is the basis of psychotherapy. In 1879, Wilhelm Wundt opened the first psychological laboratory in Germany, where he studied the mind primarily by looking at perception–a key factor in traumatization. Sigmund Freud's version of psychotherapy in the 19th and early 20th century was groundbreaking as it approached the treatment of the taboo subjects of incest and war neurosis (Morris, 1982). As scientific research expanded the understanding of the human mind and emotion, the mental heath professions moved away from relying on psychodynamic psychoanalysis. According to Roth and Fonagy (1996), in 1986, Alan Kazdin documented the use of over 400 therapeutic approaches by psychotherapists to help clients improve their quality of life (p. 3). Therapists, doctors, counselors, researchers and other practitioners have attempted to help patients mitigate symptoms and reduce their own distress by employing various techniques, methods, strategies, and procedures, such as cognitive-behavioral therapy, Gestalt, group or family therapy, Eye Movement Desensitization and Reprocessing (EMDR), narrative therapy, music, nature, Critical Incident Stress Management (CISM), art, drama, labyrinth walking, ceremonies, meditation, body movement, and/or flooding. These techniques allow survivors, in turn, to dissect painful memories, explore feelings, re-evaluate thinking styles and beliefs, and reduce symptoms of acute stress or more complicated Posttraumatic Stress Disorder (PTSD).

The traumatic experiences of combat veterans, holocaust survivors, crime victims, refugees, the chronically/terminally ill, as well as disaster responders and caregivers have led to the present version of PTSD in the *Diagnostic and Statistical Manual of Mental Disorders* (DSM-IV) of the American Psychiatric Association (1994). The manual describes PTSD as occurring subsequent to experiencing, witnessing, or the perception of a traumatic event with symptoms that include reliving the event or frightening elements of it (nightmares, flashbacks, intrusive thoughts); avoidance of memories, places, and social situations that are reminiscent of the event; emotional numbing; and hyper-vigilance.

OVERVIEW

The articles in this volume focus on techniques, which are innovative to the traumatology field. Given the breadth of work being done around the world to address the imprint that trauma leaves on individual salubriousness, documenting the successes of these techniques is a significant step in adding to the literature as well as to options practitioners have to facilitate survivors' resiliency. These new techniques described by their respective authors are designed specifically to mitigate or remove the symptoms of PTSD or acute distress from victims, survivors, and caregivers. (Although the techniques may be useful with other disorders, this will not be discussed in this volume.) Some of these innovative techniques are sometimes referred to as "power therapies" since they are fast-acting and foster resiliency.

A more detailed discussion on PTSD Motivation Enhancement Group, Residential Treatment, school-based intervention, Forensic Examination, Thought Field Therapy (TFT), Emotional Freedom Technique (EFT), Traumatic Incident Reduction (TIR), humor, art therapy, Virtual Reality therapy, and technological treatment enhancements is included. These techniques were incorporated and discussed in this volume because of their unique approach to treating trauma survivors or for their groundbreaking style.

In "Addressing Readiness to Change PTSD with a Brief Intervention: A Description of the PTSD Motivation Enhancement Group," Ronald T. Murphy and Craig S. Rosen set the tone for approaching complex PTSD in combat veterans who are ambivalent or even resistant to change at Veterans' Affairs (VA) Medical Center programs. The PTSD Motivation Enhancement Group described in this article, as a brief intervention, gets participants focused on their needs to change and the obstacles that are in the way.

The purpose of Walter Busuttil's "The Development of a 90-Day Residential Program for the Treatment of Complex Posttraumatic Stress Disorder" is to describe an inpatient program in East Sussex, England that treats veterans who were exposed to multiple and long-term traumatic incidents. The program incorporates an assessment phase, a highly structured work schedule, and follow-up.

In "How Schools Respond to Traumatic Events: Debriefing Interventions and Beyond," Mary Beth Williams describes how, as former school social worker for Falls Church City Public Schools in Virginia, she used Critical Incident Stress Management (CISM) techniques to help students cope with the September 11, 2001, terrorist attack on the

Pentagon and the subsequent Washington, DC area snipers. The guidelines Williams espouses are an expansion of conventional knowledge on crisis intervention. She also explores issues surrounding roles and planning, transmission and dissemination of information, and intervention.

In "The Forensic Examination of Posttraumatic Stress Disorder," Chrys J. Harris recognizes the ever increasing presences of PTSD in the American Judicial system as a mitigating circumstance in criminal and civil litigation. The need for accuracy and proof in a court of law adds a complicating variable to identifying perceived stressors and diagnosing PTSD. Thus, the reliance on expert witnesses to provide this evidence has grown. In this article, Harris describes a six-step methodology for conducting a forensic exam that defines parameters for examiners.

In "Thought Field Therapy: Working Through Traumatic Stress Without the Overwhelming Responses," Robert L. Bray explains the Thought Field Therapy (TFT) facilitation process. This technique, developed by Roger Callahan over the last 25 years, relies on physiology and accessing meridian treatment points in the body through tapping (much like acupuncture). Once a survivor identifies an issue and its associated level of upset, the facilitator applies the TFT algorithms until the level of upset has dissipated. TFT does not necessarily require an actual accounting of events. Its process is safe and either works or does not work. Therapists can also use TFT as a means of conducting self-care, which is often overlooked by many mental health professionals.

In "Emotional Freedom Techniques: A Safe Treatment Intervention for Many Trauma Based Issues," Garry A. Flint, Willem Lammers, and Deborah G. Mitnick describe a unique technique. Emotional Freedom Techniques (EFT) are a modification of Callahan's TFT. EFT techniques also rely on accessing meridian points in the body. The authors describe EFT as an adjunct to the Critical Incident Stress Reduction debriefing process.

Frank A. Gerbode describes Traumatic Incident Reduction (TIR) as an approach to trauma resolution in his article, "Traumatic Incident Reduction: A Person-Centered, Client-Titrated Exposure Technique." Its primary principle is to identify repressed painful memories and review them in a safe and structured manner. The repeated reviewing of traumatic memories allows the survivor to reduce or eliminate the power those memories hold.

In "The Humor of Trauma Survivors: Its Application in a Therapeutic Milieu" Jacqueline Garrick examines what humor means to Vietnam veterans and how it can be used as a coping mechanism. She defines humor and explains its applicability to the treatment process. Since trauma survivors are sometimes uncomfortable with their sense of humor, not wanting to appear as if the trauma could be minimized, they are often resistant to admitting that they see anything from a humorous perspective. Garrick describes how to engage clients appropriately by using their sense of humor as a coping tool and how to recognize when humor is inappropriate and misdirecting.

The foundation for "Art Speaks in Healing Survivors of War: The Use of Art Therapy in Treating Trauma Survivors," by Barbara Ann Baker, was a group therapy project for Bosnian War refugees settling in Chicago. The project's goal was to foster communication between clients and practitioners who did not speak the same language and clients whose culture did not value the therapeutic process. The primary activity for these refugees was the sewing of a quilt that depicted their lives in Bosnia before and during the fighting. This helped the women talk about their lives and experiences with each other and to build a new support system in the United States.

In "Virtual Reality Exposure for Veterans with Posttraumatic Stress Disorder" by David J. Ready, Stacey Pollack, Barbara Olasov Rothbaum, and Renato D. Alarcon, the authors describe Virtual Reality Exposure (VRE) as an exposure based therapy that uses technology to desensitize Vietnam veterans diagnosed with PTSD. Interjecting the virtual reality technology and equipment into the therapeutic process allows veterans undergoing treatment at the Atlanta (GA) VA Medical Center to use repeated imaginal reliving of traumatic events to assist processing of those memories. The authors detail how they introduce the Virtual Reality equipment into the therapeutic sessions, equipment operation, and research outcomes.

The final article, "Technologies to Lessen the Distress of Autism" by Ron Oberleitner, James Ball, Dan Gillette, Robert Naseef, and B. Hudnall Stamm, is a landmark documentation of the traumatic stress that families with autistic children face and how technology can reach into their isolated world and lend support and assistance. The technologies utilized in this article include telehealth, distance education, information technology, video-conferencing, and computer software with the goal of providing peer support and professional assistance to parents and their children during a crisis and to improve long-term coping skills.

While there are potentially many other techniques yet to be explored, the ones presented in this volume are the current cutting edge interventions in the field of traumatology. Further study and documentation of these techniques and others will determine the degree to which they will help those who have experienced life's worst injuries to recover, find new meaning, integrate experiences, and reach for new hopes and happiness.

REFERENCES

American Psychological Association. (1994). *Diagnostic and statistical manual of mental disorders* (4th ed.). Washington, DC: Author.

Morris, C. G. (1982). *Psychology: An introduction.* Englewood Cliffs, NJ: Prentice-Hall, Inc.

Roth, A., & Fonagy, P. (1996). *What works for whom: A critical review of psychotherapy research.* New York: Guilford Press.

Addressing Readiness to Change PTSD with a Brief Intervention: A Description of the PTSD Motivation Enhancement Group

Ronald T. Murphy
Craig S. Rosen

SUMMARY. Poor response to PTSD treatment and the disorder's chronicity among combat veterans may at least partly be due to ambivalence about the need to change PTSD symptoms and related problems. The PTSD Motivation Enhancement (ME) Group described in this article was developed to address problem acknowledgement among veterans in treatment for PTSD. This manualized, brief therapy intervention is conceptually based on the Stages of Change and draws on Motivational Interviewing techniques. The goal of the PTSD ME Group is to help patients make decisions about the need to change any behaviors and coping styles not previously recognized as problematic so that patients will perceive PTSD intervention components as more relevant, thereby fostering greater engagement in treatment and more adaptive post-treatment coping. The authors discuss theory and research findings related to

---

Address correspondence to: Ronald T. Murphy, Department of Psychology, Dillard University, Dent Hall, 2601 Gentilly Boulevard, New Orleans, LA 70122.

[Haworth co-indexing entry note]: "Addressing Readiness to Change PTSD with a Brief Intervention: A Description of the PTSD Motivation Enhancement Group." Murphy, Ronald T., and Craig S. Rosen. Co-published simultaneously in *Journal of Aggression, Maltreatment & Trauma* (The Haworth Maltreatment & Trauma Press, an imprint of The Haworth Press, Inc.) Vol. 12, No. 1/2, 2006, pp. 7-28; and: *Trauma Treatment Techniques: Innovative Trends* (ed: Jacqueline Garrick, and Mary Beth Williams) The Haworth Maltreatment & Trauma Press, an imprint of The Haworth Press, Inc., 2006, pp. 7-28. Single or multiple copies of this article are available for a fee from The Haworth Document Delivery Service [1-800-HAWORTH, 9:00 a.m. - 5:00 p.m. (EST). E-mail address: docdelivery@haworthpress.com].

7

the group, the structure and content of the intervention, and important clinical issues to consider when implementing the group. *[Article copies available for a fee from The Haworth Document Delivery Service: 1-800-HAWORTH. E-mail address: <docdelivery@haworthpress.com> Website: <http://www.HaworthPress.com>* © 2006 by The Haworth Press, Inc. All rights reserved.]

KEYWORDS. Veterans, PTSD, motivation, treatment

Combat-related posttraumatic stress disorder (PTSD) has been labeled a chronic disorder, especially among Vietnam veterans (Bremner, Southwick, Darnell, & Charney, 1996; Zlotnick, Warshaw, Shea, Allsworth, Pearlstein, & Keller, 1999). Although PTSD treatment can be effective (Foa, Keane, & Friedman, 2000; Sherman, 1998), several studies of combat veterans have found little change in PTSD symptoms following intensive treatment (Fontana & Rosenheck, 1997; Johnson, Rosenheck, Fontana, Lubin, Charney, & Southwick, 1996). Consequently, many programs treating chronic and complicated cases of PTSD have shifted from a symptom reduction model towards a "rehabilitation model," which tries to maximize patients' coping skills (Mellman, Kutcher, Santiago, & David, 1999).

Poor response to PTSD treatment and the chronicity of the disorder may at least partly be due to ambivalence about changing PTSD symptoms and related problems (Murphy, Cameron, Sharp, & Ramirez, 1999). In our experience implementing coping-focused treatments such as conflict resolution training, emotion management, and cognitive restructuring, veterans with PTSD often seemed reluctant to use new skills or give up old ways of coping. Externalization, minimization, and, more importantly, justification of trauma-based coping strategies and beliefs often resulted in patients not feeling the need or responsibility for significantly altering their behavior.

Despite negative consequences, trauma-based perceptions and strategies for coping with safety and interpersonal interactions often feel "right" or appropriate to trauma victims because of their experiences. For example, PTSD patients may view hypervigilance and isolation as effective and justifiable ways of reducing distress and ensuring safety rather than as "symptoms," as labeled by treatment providers. Anger is another example of how patients with PTSD can externalize, minimize, or justify a symptom (Chemtob, Novaco, Hamada, & Gross, 1997; Novaco & Chemtob, 1998). Many treatment-seeking combat veterans are tired of both being angry and the consequences of their anger (e.g., physical damage due to violence, family problems, and legal difficulties). Although such patients come into treatment reporting "anger problems," their view of the problem is often different from that of the therapist. The therapist may assume that patients understand their anger-related behavior as an overreaction to a current situation based on past experiences. In contrast, the patient often firmly sees his anger as a normal response to any interaction with what they view as a hostile, provocative world full of people who are careless, unaware of danger, uncaring, and threatening (DiGiuseppe, 1995; DiGiuseppe, Tafrate, & Eckhardt, 1994). We have frequently heard PTSD-diagnosed veterans say that "the average guy is stupid" with regard to trust or potential harm in the day-to-day world.

Treatment staff and patients are often unaware of how their differing assumptions impact the therapeutic alliance. Treatment providers often label patients' lack of practice or use of coping tools as resistance or symptom chronicity, attributing this to a personality trait of denial or oppositionality, IQ problems, psychodynamic defenses, bad attitude, or a general fear of change. Even if therapists and clients agree on what problems the client is facing, they may have two opposite views as to the cause of the problems and what needs to be changed (Newman, 1994). In our experience in the Veteran's Affairs (VA) PTSD treatment system, treatment providers have often experienced some PTSD patients as resistant, distrustful, and externalizing with regard to their difficulties (McBride & Markos, 1994; Zaslov, 1994). In the past, viewing treatment resistance as a personality or attitude problem inherent among veterans with PTSD led to the implementation of therapeutic community techniques that included confrontation or "attack therapy" as the preferred way of dealing with the perceived resistance. Such confrontational approaches, which have been used with substance abusers, batterers, and other populations, conflict with the need to establish empathy and a climate of safety within which trauma issues can be addressed (Murphy & Baxter, 1997; Nace, 1988; Newman, 1994). In our view, it is critical to avoid blaming trauma survivors for difficulties with distrust and avoidance, both symptoms of PTSD.

A STAGES OF CHANGE APPROACH TO PTSD SYMPTOMS AND RELATED PROBLEMS

We therefore began to consider resistance, ambivalence about change, and symptom chronicity among veterans with PTSD within the Transtheoretical Model, particularly the Stages of Change (Prochaska & Di-Clemente, 1983). The Transtheoretical Model assumes that modifiable beliefs about the need to change, rather than personality traits of denial or negative attitude, underlie the behavioral change process and response to treatment. The Stages of Change conceptualization describes five stages associated with different beliefs about the need to change and actions towards change. These stages include lack of awareness that a problem exists (Precontemplation), ambivalence about the need to change (Contemplation), taking initial steps toward change (Preparation), engagement in efforts to change (Action), and maintaining change (Maintenance). A key assumption in the Transtheoretical Model is that different psychoeducational or therapeutic techniques are needed at each stage to help individuals resolve questions about the need or ability to change that behavior and move to the next stage.

The model has most often been applied to smoking and substance abuse (Prochaska, DiClemente, & Norcross, 1992) but has been extended to a variety of other patient populations (Rosen, 2000), including male batterers (Daniels & Murphy, 1997; Levesque, Gelles, & Velicer, 2000). Readiness-to-change variables have been found to predict psychotherapy dropout (Brogan, Prochaska, & Prochaska, 1999; Smith, Subich, & Kalodner, 1995) and substance use (Belding, Iguchi, & Lamb, 1997; Heather, Rollnick, & Bell, 1993). Motivation enhancement interventions based on the Transtheoretical Model have been effective in reducing HIV risk behaviors (Carey, Maisto, Kalichman, Forsyth, Wright, & Johnson, 1997) and alcohol use by college students (Borsani & Carey, 2000), problem drinkers (Miller, Benefield, & Tonigan, 1993), and alcoholics high in anger (Project Match Research Group, 1998). Studies among trauma survivors have applied the transtheoretical model to readiness for change among adult survivors of child abuse (Koraleski & Larson, 1997) and safety and relationship behaviors of battered women (Feuer, Meade, Milstead, & Resick, 1999; Wells, 1998).

In a study of beliefs about the need to change PTSD-related symptoms and problems among veterans in inpatient PTSD treatment (Murphy et al., 2004), patients were asked to report any problems that they "Might Have," defined as problems that they wondered if they had or that other people told them that they had, but they disagreed. These "Might Haves" were listed separately from any problems that patients were sure that they had ("Definitely Have") or sure that they did not have ("Don't Have"). Results indicated that the patients reported a wide range of categories of PTSD symptoms and related behaviors as "Might

Have" problems, with the highest percentage of patients (48%) classifying anger as a "Might Have." Approximately one-third of the patients labeled isolation, depressive symptoms, trust, and health as a "Might Have," and about one-fourth reported conflict resolution, alcohol, communication, relationship/intimacy, restricted range of affect, and drugs as "Might Haves." Other types of PTSD-related problems (e.g., hypervigilance) were reported as "Might Haves" by 15-21% of the patients. Importantly, preliminary unreported analyses indicated that PTSD symptom severity levels as measured by the intrusions, avoidance, and hyperarousal subscales of the PTSD Checklist (PCL; Blanchard, Jones-Alexander, Buckley, & Forneris, 1996; Weathers, Litz, Herman, Huska, & Keane, 1993) did not differ between groups of patients who acknowledged definitely having a particular PTSD-related problem and those who did not. Another study of combat PTSD patients entering treatment with severe histories of anger and alcohol problems (Rosen et al., 2001) found these patients varied markedly in their awareness of and commitment to changing these problems.

We have adapted the Stages of Change for conceptualizing readiness to change PTSD symptoms, related behaviors and cognitions, and common comorbid conditions (see Table 1). This model includes identification of the specific intervention necessary to move an individual up to the next stage of readiness to change, or belief about the need to change. We have emphasized the conceptualization of the cognitive state of an individual in the form of a question that is unique to each stage, with particular interventions best suited for helping an individual answer that question (Miller, 1985; Miller & Rollnick, 1991; Prochaska & DiClemente, 1983). For any particular problem behavior, individuals in the Precontemplation stage do not believe that they have a problem (i.e., "What problem?"). Here, education about what constitutes a problem (e.g., hypervigilance, substance abuse, or PTSD in general) helps individuals move to the second stage, Contemplation. In this stage, individuals may begin to consider the need for change (i.e., "Do I need to change?"). Decisional balance techniques and comparison of one's behavior to population norms would be applicable for individuals at this stage to help resolve ambivalence about the need to change. Once convinced of the need to change, individuals taking some initial steps toward change may still be doubtful about their ability to complete the change process (i.e., "Can I change?"). Peer modeling and mastery experiences are helpful in the Preparation stage in building self-efficacy and promoting hope for change. The final stages are Action, in which individuals are actively making behavior changes, and Maintenance, in which they are doing what is necessary to

TABLE 1. Stage of Change Model for PTSD (after Prochaska, DiClemente et al., and Miller, Rollnick et al.)

Stage	Description	Question	Intervention
Precontemplation	Person is not considering or does not want to change a particular behavior	"What problem?"	• Education about PTSD *in general*
Contemplation	Person is certainly thinking about changing a behavior	"Do I need to change?"	• Pro's & Con's • Comparison to Norms
Preparation	Person is seriously considering and planning to change a behavior and has taken steps towards change	"Can I change?"	• Education about how therapy works • Expose to successful peers • Mastery experiences
Action	Person actively doing things to change or modify behavior	"How do I change?"	• Skill-building • Homework • Practice, role-play
Maintenance	Person continues to maintain behavioral change until it becomes permanent	"How do I keep change?"	• Lifestyle change • Continue support • Relapse prevention

maintain the behavioral change. Skill-building, practice, reinforcement, and relapse prevention are best implemented in these latter stages.

Within the Motivational Interviewing and Stages of Change frameworks, resistance is due to factors such as a lack of awareness of or sensitivity to negative consequences, the presence of emotional, cognitive, or practical roadblocks to change, and the perception of problem behaviors or consequences as normative. PTSD patients' perceptions about what is normal with regard to problems such as aggressiveness, emotional expression, mistrust, hypervigilance, violence, and substance use may be based on early childhood experiences, military training, warzone experiences, and post-military lifestyle or traumatic incidents. In addition, veterans with PTSD have often chosen partners and friends who reinforce the acceptability of isolation, conflict, emotional masking, and hypervigilance. This conceptualization can help therapists to understand patients' unwillingness to acknowledge a problem and to avoid using labels like "denial" or "not ready to change."

DEVELOPMENT OF THE PTSD MOTIVATION ENHANCEMENT GROUP

As we began to reconceptualize our patients' difficulties in engagement in and utilization of treatment within the readiness-to-change model, we proceeded to develop and implement a brief therapy group, the PTSD Motivation Enhancement (ME) Group (Murphy, Rosen, Cameron, & Thompson, 2002). Our description of this group is followed by preliminary data supporting its potential value in enhancing patients' readiness for change. It is important to emphasize, however, that randomized control studies of the group have not been completed, and so conclusive statements about the group's effectiveness in motivating patients to change PTSD symptoms and related behaviors await further research.

The PTSD ME Group is conceptually based on the Stages of Change and draws on interventions from the literature on Motivational Interviewing techniques (Miller, 1985; Miller & Rollnick, 1991). The group targets any PTSD symptom or related problem behavior (e.g., anger, hypervigilance, owning weapons, depression, substance use, smoking, and other health behaviors) that patients report ambivalence about changing or feel no need to change. The goal of the group is to help patients make decisions about the need to change any behaviors, coping styles, or beliefs not previously recognized as problematic in order to increase patient engagement in treatment and promote adaptive post-treatment coping. In other words, the group is intended to help patients shift from the Precontemplation or Contemplation stages to Preparation or Action with regard to specific problems they previously dismissed or minimized. The seven-session group is designed to meet the needs of managed-care environments that require manualized brief treatments that have measurable outcomes, with built-in program evaluation and assessment of patient satisfaction.

It is important to emphasize that the PTSD ME Group is intended to be a supplement to PTSD treatment programs rather than a "stand alone" treatment. This intervention is intended to enhance clients' active participation in direct PTSD treatment programs, particularly those aiming at symptom amelioration by means of cognitive restructuring, coping skills training, and direct therapeutic exposure. The desired outcome of participation in the PTSD ME Group is increased patient engagement in therapeutic tasks and skills rehearsal, which in turn promote changes in symptoms and adaptive functioning.

Structure and Content of the PTSD ME Group

Rationale

In the first part of every group session, group leaders present the rationale and the purpose of the PTSD ME Group to the participants. The rationale presented is that post-treatment relapse to PTSD symptoms or related difficulties may not be due to inadequate treatment or "unfixable" patients, but rather to unacknowledged problems that lead to gradual or sudden return to old coping styles. For example, social isolation and excessive alcohol use often lead to disconnection from support, poor judgement, and rumination, resulting further in depression, increased hypervigilance, intrusive thoughts, anger, and loss of control. As presented to group participants, the purpose of the group is to help patients make decisions about problems that they *might* have with regard to whether or not behavioral change is needed for a particular behavior or belief. More specifically, the goal is to help patients decide whether these behaviors or problems they "Might Have" are either definitely or definitely not a problem requiring change. A clear distinction is drawn between problems listed as "Might Have" and behaviors and cognitions that they definitely are convinced they need to change. The reasons why it might be useful to make decisions about problems they might or might not have are elicited from the group and expanded upon by the group leaders. Thus, the ultimate goal for patients is to avoid getting blindsided by unacknowledged problems following discharge.

Therapeutic Mindset

The PTSD ME Group is as much a mindset as a set of specific techniques. Our approach is informed by key principles of motivational interviewing (Miller & Rollnick, 1991). These include establishing empathy, highlighting discrepancies between patient's own goals and behavior, avoiding argumentation, rolling with resistance, and supporting self-efficacy. The therapist's role is explicitly as a consultant who provides input to patients' decisions rather than as an expert who bestows his or her own conclusions. This Socratic stance is consistent with the social psychology literature showing that encouraging people to weigh and integrate new information produces more enduring attitude change than encouraging people to simply trust an expert's authority (Petty & Cacioppo, 1984). Although the PTSD ME Group involves highly structured exercises, these exercises are explicitly designed to allow clients autonomy to choose which problems to focus on, grapple with decisions, and conclude for themselves whether the results of a given session indicate they need to change.

In implementing the group, group leaders should follow the overall approach recommended by Newman (1994) and Miller and colleagues (Miller, 1985; Miller & Rollnick, 1991): being objective and non-confrontational, and always using empathic listening techniques to address patients' responses, no matter how oppositional they might seem. We have found that many clinicians, regardless of experience, have difficulty taking a non-confrontational stance with provocative and externalizing patients. Yet maintaining an objective and supportive stance is especially important when working with angry and provocative patients (DiGiuseppe et al., 1994; Murphy & Baxter, 1997). The importance of maintaining empathy is underscored by the research finding that therapist empathy and client report of the working alliance is the most consistent predictor of psychotherapy outcome (Horvath & Luborsky, 1993; Horvath & Symonds, 1991; Miller et al., 1993).

General Structure

The sequence of groups was designed in a rolling admissions context where participants may enter the group at any module. The group protocol consists of seven group sessions: six sessions with four separate group modules (two modules are repeated) and a seventh session repeating the first group attended (see Table 2). This seventh session was added because some veterans can be disoriented or have some difficulty understanding group content in their first session after entering treatment. To further accommodate the effects of rolling admissions and the extent of memory and attention deficit in aging veteran populations, behavioral learning principles of repetition and rehearsal are used by reviewing the purpose, rationale, and format of the group during the first half of each of the seven group sessions. In this review period, time is given to individualized identification of "Might Have" problems. This review is accomplished by asking questions of the group and allowing more experienced members to answer, thereby educating and acculturating the newcomers. The second half of each session consists of discussion of module-specific tools that will assist patients in deciding whether or not problems that they might have are behaviors they need to change. Group leaders follow a manualized protocol, but the format is interactive and makes extensive use of a whiteboard and patient worksheets.

TABLE 2. PTSD ME Group Session Outline

Session	Group Module	Tasks/Material Covered
Session 1	Group Overview	- Review purpose and potential value of the group - Generate list of problems Definitely Have, Might Have, Don't Have
Sessions 2 & 3	Comparison to the Average Guy	- Review purpose and potential value of the group - Generate list of problems Definitely Have, Might Have, Don't Have - Patients compare their behavior to estimated age-appropriate "norms" in order to help them judge how problematic their behavior might be
Sessions 4 & 5	Pro's & Con's	- Review purpose and potential value of the group - Generate list of problems Definitely Have, Might Have, Don't Have - Decision balance techniques used to help patients decide about the need to change "Might Be A Problem" behaviors which they agree they do, but are not sure are actually problematic
Session 6	Roadblocks	- Review purpose and potential value of the group - Generate list of problems Definitely Have, Might Have, Don't Have - Identify fears, cognitive distortions, and stereotype beliefs that prevent problem identification
Session 7	In rolling admission context, patient repeats first group attended	

Group Content

A key part of the group is having patients generate a list of problem areas that might be a problem for them. This process occurs in the first half of every session, following the general review of rationale and purpose. At that time, patients fill out a worksheet that is divided into three columns: "Definitely Have," "Might Have," or "Definitely Don't Have" (see Figure 1). The "Might Have" column is further divided into two categories: "A Problem You Have Wondered If You Have" and "A Problem Other People Say You Have (But You Disagree)." We have defined "Might Have" problems in these two ways to elicit not only problem areas that they have considered as possibly needing change (i.e., on which they are in Contemplation stage), but also problems that they might be unaware of or unwilling to change (i.e., Precontemplation stage). The goal is for patients to eventually sort items listed under "Might Have" into "Definitely Have" or "Definitely Don't Have."

Group Modules

In the first module (Session 1), "Group Overview," the purpose and potential value of the group is reviewed in detail. Time is also used for reviewing the worksheet on which patients identify problems they "Might Have." The second module, "Comparison to the Average Guy" (Sessions 2 & 3), is aimed at helping patients compare their behavior to estimated age-appropriate but non-PTSD "norms" in order to help them judge how problematic their behavior might be. Behaviors are catego-

FIGURE 1. "Form #1" Worksheet for PTSD ME Group

	MIGHT HAVES		
Problems You DEFINITELY HAVE	Problems you might have: You have wondered if you have	Problems you might have: Problems other people say you have but you disagree	Problems You DEFINITELY DON'T HAVE

rized along a range including "Average," "Moderate Problem," and "Extreme Problem." Three dimensions are used to assess behavior at each of these levels: frequency, severity of consequences, and purpose. Group leaders guide members in analyzing what a particular behavior would look like at each of the three levels on each of the three dimensions. For example, if hypervigilance was the behavior selected, group leaders would first elicit a description of normative levels of safety awareness, including checking door locks at night and installing motion-sensitive lights outside. Minor consequences of this normative level would be mild other than the cost of the lights, with the purpose being to feel reasonably safe. Next, there is discussion about what constitutes a moderate level of excessive caution or security-consciousness, such as checking doors twice and getting an attack dog, with consequences including more time and money invested, and intimidating people with the dog. The purpose here begins to take on more of an anxiety-reduction role. Extreme levels of caution, or hypervigilance, may include checking the perimeter of the house throughout the night, keeping a gun under the bed, having multiple weapons, and setting booby traps. At this level, consequences are increased time and energy spent and risk to children, with the purpose of these behaviors involving feelings of survival and a sense of a "life or death" situation.

In the third module, "Pros & Cons" (Sessions 4 & 5), decision balance techniques are reviewed and practiced to help patients decide about the need to change "Might Have" behaviors that they acknowledge doing, but they are not sure are actually problematic. In this simple but effective technique, patients weigh the advantages and disadvantages of various PTSD symptoms and related behaviors, such as gun ownership, hypervigilance (e.g., "setting perimeters"), needing to be in control, a general mistrust of others, social isolation, or continued substance use.

The final module, "Roadblocks" (Session 6), focuses on beliefs or feelings that make it difficult to even consider the need to change. Common roadblocks to considering change include fears, cognitive distortions, and inaccurate stereotypes about what it means to have a problem. Fears of being overwhelmed by problems or being rejected if problems are acknowledged are some of the roadblocks reviewed. Also, there may be cognitive distortions and errors, such as "all or nothing thinking" (e.g., "If I admit to having one more problem, I will have to acknowledge being a complete failure") or blaming of others. Stereotypes of what it means to be an alcoholic (e.g., the town drunk, homeless) or a psychiatric patient ("another crazy Vietnam veteran") can cause reluctance to admit to an alcohol problem or avoidance of psychotherapy.

The group generates a variety of possible roadblocks and participants are instructed to fill out their worksheet to identify and list only those that apply to them. Psychological issues related to shame and guilt frequently arise in the context of this group. The collaborative process provides a supportive context in which veterans can normalize and experience the universality of their feelings, and recognize personal roadblocks to considering the need for change.

Group Process

For successful implementation of the PTSD ME Group, it is important to promote interaction and active participation during the group sessions so that patients gain a sense of ownership of the therapeutic process and their decision-making (Newman, 1994; Rosen & Sharp, 1998). Active engagement in group tasks may also help participants to better comprehend, remember, and apply the concepts and information learned. Although the facilitator provides an overall structure to the discussion, patients are encouraged to verbalize their responses so that more active, insightful, or adept group members can serve as role models and facilitate observational learning with regard to the practical aspects of group participation. This also creates an atmosphere of openness and helps prompt anxious or distrustful members to participate. To enhance this process, we encourage facilitators to ask group members to provide answers to questions from fellow participants. Most importantly, patients are encouraged to use the process to draw their own conclusions about whether they need to change any particular behavior. This helps reduce patient reactance and oppositional responding, which is especially important given that many patients have been in treatment settings where ambivalence or disagreement with therapists has been met with confrontation, being labeled as "not ready for treatment" or "resistant," or threats of discharge.

THE PTSD ME GROUP: CLINICAL CONSIDERATIONS

Selecting Appropriate Patients for the PTSD ME Group

The PTSD ME Group has been implemented most extensively with veterans whose PTSD is long-standing and arose from multiple traumatic experiences, sometimes over their entire lifespan. These patients often have a complicated symptom picture with many varied PTSD symptoms and related problems. The PTSD ME Group, therefore, was designed to address patients experiencing a variety of problems, with the assumption that there will be variation in readiness to change across different PTSD symptoms and other problems. The PTSD ME Group, then, may not be appropriate for individuals with a recent, single-incident trauma, for example, with a circumscribed set of trauma symptoms and less general life dysfunction. Some of the PTSD ME Group techniques, however, may be helpful for such a patient who seems ambivalent or unaware of the need to change certain coping behaviors or beliefs related to the traumatic event.

As with any group intervention, candidates for participation in the PTSD ME Group should be able to tolerate group process, cooperate with peers, and contribute to an atmosphere of physical and emotional safety in the group. We have found that patients who were unable to form bonds with veteran peers, especially in an inpatient setting, did not find the group useful and could be disruptive despite our best intervention efforts. More specific to the PTSD ME Group, some patients who refuse to consider that they can be unaware of or ambivalent about the need to change any behavior or belief do not get much benefit from the group. This includes patients who have a strong "all or nothing" cognitive style. For some of these patients, review of the PTSD ME Group rationale, taking an empathic approach, and discussion of possible roadblocks to problem acknowledgement helps patients take advantage of the group. In addition, having the patient identify "all or nothing thinking" as a possible problem can be beneficial.

Troubleshooting Difficult Situations

In any group treatment, participants may become oppositional, negative, or disruptive. In the PTSD ME Group in particular, this has taken the form of attacks on the value of thinking about possible unacknowledged problems and anger about the perceived lack of relationship of the group to coping with PTSD. In addition, we have often had veterans strongly express that the PTSD ME Group does not address their betrayal by the government, and they want the therapists to allow discussion of what they see as the critical issue in the treatment of their distress. We have found it helpful, consistent with the mindset discussion above, to avoid labeling a difficult patient as disruptive, and instead conceptualize the situation as arising from the patient not yet understanding the rationale and potential value of the group. Also, patients who have difficulty grasping the content of the group may be expressing their frustration in a more externalizing manner. We have found that some aspects of the PTSD ME Group can be difficult to comprehend at first, including the "Comparison to the Average Guy" module, the "Might Have" concept, and how this concept relates to the goal of the group. Further, some patients are overwhelmed by the volume of information presented, especially patients with poor cognitive functioning related to substance use.

In general, some potential problems can be averted by making sure that the rationale and goal of the group have been carefully presented at the outset, particularly that symptom exacerbation after treatment may be related to the patient "missing something" in their understanding of their distress. We also will acknowledge that being in therapy can be difficult, and we encourage patients to not let all their hard work go to waste by letting unresolved issues or strong feelings interfere with their engagement in treatment. As always, reflective listening to patient concerns is invaluable in gaining patient trust and cooperation, and actually is most effective when those concerns have been expressed negatively. In addition, questions or expressed frustration about the content of the group can usually be reframed by the therapist as helpful to the group (e.g., acknowledging that the patient's questions or concerns are understandable and give the leaders an opportunity to clarify points that can be hard to understand). This is important because we feel that too many therapists overestimate their ability to use jargon-free language that is consistent with the average person's educational background and level of psychological mindedness. For patients who are becoming excessively hostile, limit-setting is necessary, although best done by calmly but firmly clarifying what behaviors or phrases are unacceptable. Even at this point, patients often respond well to explanations about why the limits exist (e.g., to preserve therapeutic process, assist patient in goals of self-control and communication, etc). Appropriate confrontation in therapy can include discussion with a patient about how their behavior relates to their goals, values, and reasons for coming to treatment.

EVALUATING PATIENT PROGRESS IN THE PTSD ME GROUP

Assessing patient response to the PTSD ME Group can give therapists more specific guidance to patients in utilizing the group effectively, provide some positive feedback to patients about their participation, and prompt therapists to consider modifications in how they are running the group. We recommend assessing changes in problem awareness and ambivalence, and clinical indicators of patient change.

Tracking Changes in Problem Ambivalence or Awareness

At the end of every group, each participant is asked to list on the Weekly Review Form any problems that they identified as "Might Have" during the course of that particular session. In addition, patients are asked to report if they re-classified any previously identified "Might Haves" as "Definitely A Problem" or "Definitely Not A Problem" at any time during that group session. These data can be kept for each patient to track individual changes in beliefs about the need to change the "Might Haves" over the course of the group.

Clinical Indicators

The PTSD ME group is intended to improve patients' symptoms and functioning by increasing active participation in other components of PTSD treatment. Useful measures of patient progress, then, would be indices of patient's engagement in other PTSD treatment program components. This could include data from other treating clinicians on patient completion of therapy and homework tasks, skills rehearsal, reports of real-world coping skills use, and clinician ratings of therapy engagement.

PTSD ME GROUP: INTEGRATION INTO PROGRAMS

The PTSD ME Group, as a brief therapy intervention, was designed to be used as an adjunctive treatment within a larger treatment program. We discuss below three models for how this group can be integrated into a more comprehensive PTSD treatment plan: as a concurrent adjunct treatment, as a preliminary phase of treatment, and as a module within ongoing semi-structured group therapy. We also discuss relative advantages of open versus closed groups.

Concurrent Adjunct Treatment

In our first major trial at the National Center for PTSD in Menlo Park, the PTSD ME Group was run concurrently with all other treatment components in a 60-day inpatient VA PTSD program. An advantage of this approach is that it provides a forum for continually working through ambivalence issues that may ebb and flow over the course of treatment, and for integrating feedback patients receive from other milieu members. However, an important disadvantage of running the group over the same time period as other groups and activities is that patients may be introduced to various coping skills before they have time to decide which elements they need. For example, given that almost 50% of patients may be ambivalent about anger being a problem for them, a number of participants in anger management groups may be less motivated to learn, practice, or use new ways of dealing with anger.

Preliminary Phase of Treatment

Having the PTSD ME Group near the beginning of treatment may further enhance the therapeutic process, when patients are developing goals and objectives. This is the model used in the PTSD Outpatient Clinic at the New Orleans VA Medical Center, where PTSD ME Group is currently used as part of the second of five phases of treatment. After veterans complete four weekly PTSD Education Group sessions, patients then move to the PTSD ME Group and a case management group where they begin to identify problems, develop treatment plans, and discuss progress. This prepares patients to actively participate in the third, fourth, and fifth phases of treatment, which respectively address coping skills, developmental issues, and relapse prevention. It is hoped that placement of the PTSD ME Group in this sequence affords patients the opportunity to enter the more active phases of treatment with increased awareness of their potential difficulties and greater clarity about their personal treatment goals. An alternative to this phase approach would be to offer a two or three session version of the PTSD ME Group to patients who are considering whether or not to start or continue treatment, in order to help patients make better decisions about the need to begin involvement in therapy or engage in additional treatment components.

Treatment Module Within an Ongoing Process Group

In the VA, many PTSD patients are treated in ongoing process-oriented or supportive therapy groups. The PTSD ME Group could be used as a monthly or occasional module within such ongoing groups to help clients continually clarify their current treatment goals and priorities.

Open vs. Closed Groups

The PTSD ME Group is most simply implemented within a closed group, where all patients are introduced to the same material at the same time. However, this group has also been implemented as an open group within a treatment program with rolling admissions. Although this required more flexibility and repetition to accommodate new members, the open group format had the unexpected advantage of creating a mix of senior and new patients in the PTSD ME Group. This allowed more senior peers to act as advisors and role models for newer members of the group, which enhanced learning for both newer and senior members.

PRELIMINARY FINDINGS
ON PTSD ME GROUP EFFECTIVENESS

Findings from our uncontrolled evaluation study of the PTSD ME Group (Murphy et al., 2004) will only be briefly summarized here. Data were collected over an 18-month period from 243 inpatients that attended the PTSD ME Group during their stay in a VA PTSD treatment program. Over the course of the group, veterans on average reclassified approximately 40% of all items they initially listed as "Might Have" to either "Definitely Have" or "Definitely Don't Have." For patients who classified various problems as "Might Have," by the end of their participation in the group significantly more veterans reclassified anger, isolation, anxiety, authority, guilt, emotional masking, relationship/intimacy, smoking, and trust problems as "Definitely Have" than "Definitely Don't Have." Group participants reported high levels of satisfaction with all aspects of group content and process, and gave high ratings on helpfulness (Franklin, Murphy, Cameron, Ramirez, Sharp, & Drescher, 1999). Findings also indicated that compensation status and ethnicity were significantly related to reported frequency of problem awareness or ambivalence or changes in these variables (Murphy et al., 2000). Although definitive statements about the effectiveness of the group await controlled trials, these initial findings indicate that patients are responding to the group as predicted.

READINESS TO CHANGE
AND PTSD TREATMENT OUTCOME

The ultimate goal of participation in the PTSD ME Group is improvement of post-treatment functioning. Currently, PTSD treatment programs usually focus on teaching veterans new coping behaviors and self-talk with the aim of suppressing or replacing maladaptive behavior, cognitions, and emotions. Even many exposure-based treatments, including stress inoculation training, are based on having patients approach feared or unpleasant cues and memories without resorting to avoidance-based coping strategies. These approaches are based on the assumption that this chronic population of VA patients is ready to give up long-held styles of thinking and acting. However, patients are less likely to learn new coping behaviors or ways of thinking if they are unconvinced about the need to change any old ways of acting and thinking. If patients are not convinced that a particular reaction or behavioral response to stress is a PTSD-related problem, they may make less use of new coping tools for those problems or fail to apply newly learned skills outside the immediate treatment setting.

The ultimate goal of our ongoing research efforts is to determine if the addition of a PTSD ME Group to a PTSD treatment program results in better learning, practice, and implementation of coping skills, which in turn should produce better post-treatment functioning. We hope that this motivational enhancement intervention, although still under development, may offer a new approach for increasing the effectiveness of PTSD treatment and prompt reconsideration of current attributions for PTSD treatment failure and the disorder's chronicity among veterans. Further evolution of the PTSD ME Group and judgement of its value, practicality, and long-term impact on patient functioning will be based on the results of research and on feedback from clinicians implementing the group.

REFERENCES

Belding, M., Iguchi, M., & Lamb, R. (1997). Stages and processes of change as predictors of drug use among methadone maintenance patients. *Experimental and Clinical Psychopharmacology, 5*(1), 65-73.

Blanchard, E. B., Jones-Alexander, J., Buckley, T. C., & Forneris, C. A. (1996). Psychometric properties of the PTSD Checklist (PCL). *Behaviour Research and Therapy, 34*, 669-673.

Borsani, B., & Carey, K. B. (2000). Effects of a brief motivational intervention with college student drinkers. *Journal of Consulting and Clinical Psychology, 68*, 728-733.

Bremner, J. D., Southwick, S. M., Darnell, A., & Charney, D. S. (1996). Chronic PTSD in Vietnam combat veterans: Course of illness and substance abuse. *American Journal of Psychiatry, 153*(3), 369-375.

Brogan, M. M., Prochaska, J. O., & Prochaska, J. M. (1999). Predicting termination and continuation status in psychotherapy using the transtheoretical model. *Psychotherapy, 36*(2), 50-60.

Carey, M. P., Maisto, S. A., Kalichman, S. C., Forsyth, A. D., Wright, E. M., & Johnson, B. T. (1997). Enhancing motivation to reduce the risk of HIV infection for economically disadvantaged urban women. *Journal of Consulting and Clinical Psychology, 65*, 531-541.

Chemtob, C. M., Novaco, R. W., Hamada, R. S., & Gross, D. M. (1997). Cognitive-behavioral treatment for severe anger in posttraumatic stress disorder. *Journal of Consulting and Clinical Psychology, 65*(1), 184-189.

Daniels, J. W., & Murphy, C. W. (1997). Stages and processes of change in batterers' treatment. *Cognitive and Behavioral Practice, 4*(1), 123-145.

DiGiuseppe, R. (1995). Developing the therapeutic alliance with angry clients. In H. Kassinove (Ed.), *Anger disorders: Definition, diagnosis and treatment* (pp. 131-150). Philadelphia, PA: Taylor & Francis.

DiGiuseppe, R., Tafrate, R. & Eckhardt, C. (1994). Critical issues in the treatment of anger. *Cognitive & Behavioral Practice, 1*, 111-132.

Feuer, C., Meade, L., Milstead, M., & Resick, P. (1999, November). *The transtheoretical model applied to domestic violence survivors.* Paper presented at the annual meeting of the International Society for Traumatic Stress Studies, Miami, FL.

Foa, E. B., Keane, T. M., & Friedman, M. J. (2000). *Effective treatments for PTSD: Practice guidelines from the International Society for Traumatic Stress Studies.* New York: Guilford Press.

Fontana, A., & Rosenheck, R. (1997). Effectiveness and cost of the inpatient treatment of posttraumatic stress disorder: Comparison of three models of treatment. *American Journal of Psychiatry, 154*, 758-765.

Franklin, C. L., Murphy, R. T., Cameron, R. P., Ramirez, G., Sharp, L. D., & Drescher, K. D. (1999, November). *Perceived helpfulness of a group targeting motivation to change PTSD symptoms.* Poster session presented at the annual meeting of the International Society for Traumatic Stress Studies, Miami, FL.

Heather, N., Rollnick, S., & Bell, A. (1993). Predictive validity of the Readiness to Change questionnaire. *Addiction, 88*, 1667-1677.

Horvath, A. O., & Luborsky, L. (1993). The role of the therapeutic alliance in psychotherapy. *Journal of Consulting and Clinical Psychology, 61*, 561-573.

Horvath, A. O., & Symonds, B. D. (1991). Relation between working alliance and outcome in psychotherapy: A meta-analysis. *Journal of Counseling Psychology, 38*, 138-149.

Johnson, D. R., Rosenheck, R., Fontana, A., Lubin, H., Charney, D., & Southwick, S. (1996). Outcome of intensive inpatient treatment for combat-related posttraumatic stress disorder. *American Journal of Psychiatry, 153*(6), 771-777.

Koraleski, S. F., & Larson, L. M. (1997). A partial test of the Transtheoretical Model in therapy with adult survivors of childhood sexual abuse. *Journal of Counseling Psychology, 44*(3), 302-306.

Levesque, D. A., Gelles, R. J., & Velicer, W. F. (2000). Development and validation of a stages of change measure for men in batterer treatment. *Cognitive Therapy and Research, 24*, 175-199.

McBride, M. C., & Markos, P. A. (1994). Sources of difficulty in counselling sexual abuse victims and survivors. Special Issue: Perspectives on working with difficult clients. *Canadian Journal of Counseling, 28*(1), 83-99.

Mellman, T. A., Kutcher, G. S., Santiago, L., & David, D. (1999). Rehabilitative treatment for combat-related PTSD. *Psychiatric Services, 50,* 1363-1364.

Miller, W. R. (1985). Motivation for treatment: A review with a special emphasis on alcoholism. *Psychological Bulletin, 99,* 84-107.

Miller, W. R., Benefield, R. G., & Tonigan, J. S. (1993). Enhancing motivation for change in problem drinking: A controlled comparison of two therapist styles. *Journal of Consulting and Clinical Psychology, 61,* 455-461.

Miller, W. R., & Rollnick, S. (1991). *Motivational interviewing.* New York: Guilford.

Murphy, C. M., & Baxter, V. A. (1997). Motivating batterers to change in the treatment context. *Journal of Interpersonal Violence, 12*(4), 607-619.

Murphy, R. T., Cameron, R. P., Sharp, L., & Ramirez, G. (1999). Motivating veterans to change PTSD symptoms and related behaviors. *PTSD Clinical Quarterly, 8(2),* 32-36.

Murphy, R. T., Cameron, R. P., Sharp, L., Ramirez, G., Rosen, C., Drescher, K. et al. (2004). Readiness to change PTSD symptoms and related behaviors among veterans participating in a motivation enhancement group. *The Behavior Therapist, 27*(4), 33-36.

Murphy, R. T., Drescher, K., Sharp, L., Ramirez, G., Rosen, C., Cameron, R. P. et al. (2000, November). *Individual differences in readiness to change PTSD: Service-connection and ethnicity.* Poster session presented at annual meeting of the International Society for Traumatic Stress Studies, San Antonio, TX.

Murphy, R. T., Rosen, C. S., Cameron, R. P., & Thompson, K. E. (2002). Development of a group treatment for enhancing motivation to change PTSD symptoms. *Cognitive & Behavioral Practice, 9 (4),* 308-316.

Nace, E. P. (1988). Posttraumatic stress disorder and substance abuse: Clinical issues. In M. Galanter (Ed.), *Recent developments in alcoholism* (Vol 6., pp. 9-26). New York: Plenum.

Newman, C. F. (1994). Understanding client resistance: Methods for enhancing motivation to change. *Cognitive and Behavioral Practice, 1,* 47-69.

Novaco, R. W., & Chemtob, C. C. (1998). Anger and trauma: Conceptualization, assessment and treatment. In V. M. Follette, J. I. Ruzek, & F. R. Abueg (Eds.), *Cognitive-behavioral therapies for trauma* (pp. 162-190). New York: Guilford.

Petty, R. E., & Cacioppo, J. T. (1984). The effects of involvement on response to argument quality and quantity: Central and peripheral routes to persuasion. *Journal of Personality and Social Psychology, 46,* 69-81.

Prochaska, J. O., & DiClemente, C. C. (1983). Stages and processes of self-change in smoking: Toward an integrative model of change. *Journal of Consulting & Clinical Psychology, 40,* 432-440.

Prochaska, J. O., DiClemente, C. C., & Norcross, J. C. (1992). In search of how people change: Applications to addictive behaviors. *American Psychologist, 47,* 1102-1114.

Project Match Research Group. (1998). Matching alcoholism treatments to client heterogeneity: Project MATCH three-year drinking outcomes. *Alcoholism: Clinical and Experimental Research, 22*(6), 1300-1311.

Rosen, C. S. (2000). Is the sequencing of change processes by stage consistent across health problems? A meta-analysis. *Health Psychology, 19*, 593-604.

Rosen, C. S., Murphy, R. T., Chow, H. C., Drescher, K. D., Ramirez, G., Ruddy, R. et al. (2001). Posttraumatic stress disorder patients' readiness to change alcohol and anger problems. *Psychotherapy, 38*, 233-244.

Rosen, C. S., & Sharp, L. (1998, November). Using the Elaboration Likelihood Model (ELM) to improve motivational interventions. In R. Murphy (Chair), *Stages of change in assessment and treatment of PTSD*. Symposium conducted at the annual meeting of the International Society for Study of Traumatic Stress, Washington, DC.

Sherman, J. J. (1998). Effects of psychotherapeutic treatments for PTSD: A meta-analysis of controlled clinical trials. *Journal of Traumatic Stress, 11*(3), 413-435.

Smith, K. J., Subich, L. M., & Kalodner, C. (1995). The transtheoretical model's stages and processes of change and their relation to premature termination. *Journal of Counseling Psychology, 42*, 34-39.

Weathers, F. W., Litz, B. T., Herman, J.A., Huska, J. A., & Keane, T. M. (1993, November). *The PTSD Checklist (PCL): Reliability, validity and diagnostic utility*. Paper presented at the 9th Annual Conference of the International Society for Study of Traumatic Stress, San Antonio, TX.

Wells, M. T. (1998, November). *Assessing battered women's readiness to change: An instrument development study*. Paper presented at the annual meeting of the International Society for Traumatic Stress Studies, Washington, DC.

Zaslov, M. R. (1994). Psychology of comorbid posttraumatic stress disorder and substance abuse: Lessons from combat veterans. *Journal of Psychoactive Drugs, 26*(4), 393-400.

Zlotnick, C., Warshaw, M., Shea, M. T., Allsworth, J., Pearlstein, T., & Keller, M. B. (1999). Chronicity in posttraumatic stress disorder (PTSD) and predictors of course of co-morbid PTSD in patients with anxiety disorders. *Journal of Traumatic Stress, 12*(1), 89-100.

The Development
of a 90-Day Residential Program for the Treatment of Complex Posttraumatic Stress Disorder

Walter Busuttil

SUMMARY. Based on the author's previous work with military personnel suffering from PTSD, a 90-day residential treatment program for Complex PTSD was designed and implemented at Priory Ticehurst House Hospital. It comprises an assessment protocol, a highly structured work schedule, and day case follow-up reviews at six weeks, six months, and one year. Results of the present study suggest that the program promoted significant global improvement in terms of PTSD status, depression, and occupational and social function, with hospital admission days also reduced significantly over the follow-up period. These promising results prompt the need for empirical controlled studies in order to assess

Address correspondence to Walter Busuttil, The Priory Ticehurst House, Ticehurst, Wadhurst, East Sussex, TN5 7HU (E-mail: walterbusuttil@prioryhealthcare.com).

The author would like to acknowledge the tireless encouragement of his co-director Dr. Gordon J. Turnbull, the staff on the CPTSD ward, and especially Ms. Sue Pitman who played an important role in setting up this program. Thanks also to his wife, Dr. Angela Busuttil, clinical psychologist, for her useful critical comments, which contributed to the therapeutic approaches adopted by the program.

[Haworth co-indexing entry note]: "The Development of a 90-Day Residential Program for the Treatment of Complex Posttraumatic Stress Disorder." Busuttil, Walter. Co-published simultaneously in *Journal of Aggression, Maltreatment & Trauma* (The Haworth Maltreatment & Trauma Press, an imprint of The Haworth Press, Inc.) Vol. 12, No. 1/2, 2006, pp. 29-55; and: *Trauma Treatment Techniques: Innovative Trends* (ed: Jacqueline Garrick, and Mary Beth Williams) The Haworth Maltreatment & Trauma Press, an imprint of The Haworth Press, Inc., 2006, pp. 29-55. Single or multiple copies of this article are available for a fee from The Haworth Document Delivery Service [1-800-HAWORTH, 9:00 a.m. - 5:00 p.m. (EST). E-mail address: docdelivery@haworthpress.com].

Available online at http://www.haworthpress.com/web/JAMT
doi:10.1300/J146v12n01_03

the full efficacy of this approach in intervening with chronically ill patients suffering from Complex PTSD. *[Article copies available for a fee from The Haworth Document Delivery Service: 1-800- HAWORTH. E-mail address: <docdelivery@haworthpress.com> Website: <http://www.HaworthPress.com> © 2006 by The Haworth Press, Inc. All rights reserved.]*

KEYWORDS. Complex Posttraumatic Stress Disorder, psychiatric rehabilitation, group therapy rehabilitation programs

As a concept, Complex Posttraumatic Stress Disorder (PTSD) has been referred to and described at several points during the history of psychiatry. For example, it was described in the definition of the Concentration Camp Syndrome in the 1940s and 1950s (Chodoff, 1963; Eitinger, 1959, 1961, 1964; Thygesen, Hermann, & Willanger, 1970) and in the conceptualizations of the psychiatric effects on victims of torture (Turner & Gorst-Unsworth, 1990), crime (Kilpatrick, Saunders, & Vernonen, 1987), and rape (Burgess & Holmstrom, 1976, 1979; Burgess, Holstrom, Marmar, & Krupnick, 1980). In addition, the concept of a complex form of PTSD resulting from exposure to multiple traumas can also be found in the Palo Alto Model for the rehabilitation of Vietnam Veterans posited by Scurfield (1993) and in the Sanctuary Model for victims of multiple traumas proposed by Bloom (1997). The *Diagnostic and Statistical Manual of Mental Disorders* (DSM-IV; American Psychiatric Association, 1994) Field Trial defined Complex PTSD as having specific characteristics differentiating it from PTSD seen following exposure to single adult trauma (van der Kolk, Roth, Pelcovitz, & Mandel, 1994).

Plans for the rehabilitation of the British hostages released from Beirut in 1991 prompted research by the Royal Air Force Psychiatric Services to further investigate the effects of unrelenting, multiple trauma (Busuttil, 1993; Busuttil, Aquilina, & Busuttil, 1993; Psychiatric Division of the Royal Air Force Medical Service, 1993; Turnbull, 1992; Turnbull & Busuttil, 1992a, 1992b). For example, those subjected to this ordeal were exposed to the following traumas: (a) the subjection to pre-captivity traumatic experiences; (b) the trauma of capture itself; (c) the subjection to torture; (d) the subjection to solitary and group confinement; and (e) the experience of being denied freedom itself (Busuttil, 1993). More recently, researchers have made additional efforts to promote a better understanding of the psychiatric symptoms and behavioral changes resulting from the subjection to multiple traumas. The constellation of psychological and behavioral symptoms that can result from such experiences has been conceptualized as Complex PTSD in the resulting literature.

Judith Herman (1992, 1993), for example, suggested that a separate diagnostic category of PTSD was required to fully describe the psychiatric effects of multiple traumatic stresses. She consequently coined the concept of Disorders of Extreme Stress Not Otherwise Specified (DESNOS) and proposed its inclusion in the DSM-IV; she also presented evidence from the literature in support of her proposal. Herman highlighted a tri-dimensional model comprised of: (a) observed symptoms; (b) character traits; and (c) the vulnerability to repeated harm (of the self, inflicted by others, or inflicted to others).

Herman's proposal instigated the DSM-IV Field Trial for PTSD, which studied the relationship between the development of PTSD and a co-existent syndrome of other psychological symptoms and difficulties commonly associated with a history of exposure to extreme multiple psychological traumas (van der Kolk et al., 1994). The term Disorders of Extreme Stress (DES) was coined to describe a syndrome involving a disturbance in the following seven areas: (a) affect and impulse; (b) attention and concentration; (c) self-perception; (d) perception of perpetrator; (e) relationships with others; (f) somatic complaints; and (g) systems of meaning.

Prevalence of DES symptoms was correlated with PTSD, age of onset, and duration of the trauma in 328 psychiatric outpatients who had been subjected to multiple traumas (van der Kolk et al., 1994). The study concluded that DES described a syndrome of psychiatric disturbance related to early, chronic interpersonal trauma associated with PTSD. The combination of DES and PTSD was termed Complex PTSD. According to Bloom (1997), further work has led to an expanded understanding of this proposed syndrome. Bloom (1997) included three areas of disturbance in her working model of Complex PTSD (see Table 1). These comprise Symptoms, Character Changes, and a propensity to a Repetition of Harm. The Symptom area includes symptoms of PTSD and/or Somatic, Affective, and Dissociative symptoms. Character Changes include those governed by a sense of Control that can lead to 'traumatic bonding' in relationships, a pervading sense of fear, and other relationship difficulties, including a 'lens of extremity' leading to ambivalence between making and retaining attachments versus withdrawal from these attachments. Identity Changes are also included in this area of disturbance, with distortions in relation to self-structures. This includes an 'internalized image of stress,' a 'malignant sense of self,' and a 'fragmentation of the self.' In the final area of disturbance, a propensity to a repetition of harm is described.

TABLE 1. Mean Scores by Time

	n	CAPS-1 Symptom Intensity			CAPS-1 Occupational Function			CAPS-1 Social Function			IES Total Score			BDI			GHQ-28		
		range	Mean	SD	range	Mean	SD	range	Mean	SD	range	Mean	SD	range	Mean	SD	range	Mean	SD
T1	25	35-61	51.1	6.5	3-4	3.9	0.3	3-4	3.9	0.3	41-73	57.3	8.3	14-53	35.1	8.8	3-28	18.3	7.5
T2	24	8-58	33.1	13.2	0-4	2.3	1.5	0-4	2.0	1.3	2-75	42.5	20.1	1-49	22.9	14.0	0-28	10.5	9.6
T3	15	11-58	33.3	15.9	0-4	2.0	1.6	0-4	1.9	1.5	7-75	48.3	19.4	0-47	23.3	15.6	0-25	9.7	6.4
T4	12	6-50	28.8	13.1	0-4	2.0	1.1	0-4	1.6	0.9	10-73	39.5	17.7	0-40	24.1	11.8	0-22	12.3	6.5

Note: T1 = Pre-treatment; T2 = six weeks; T3 = six months; T4 = one year

This may include harm to the self through repeated deliberate self-harm or through faulty boundary setting (the so-called cycle of violence), harm perpetrated by others (including battery and abuse), and harm perpetrated of others where the victim becomes an abuser. It should be noted that in Bloom's rationale, overlap exists with the diagnostic criteria of Border-line Personality Disorder (BPD) as defined by the DSM-IV. This overlap relates especially to the characterological changes and a propensity to harm areas.

The model presented by Herman (1992, 1993) and elaborated on by van der Kolk et al. (1994) and Bloom (1997) had a great influence in the therapeutic approaches adopted when devising this treatment program. Bloom's (1997) rationale led to the following framework in conceptual-izing Complex PTSD. This was important in the drawing up of the psy-cho-education material covered within the program (Busuttil, 2000).

According to the recognized information processing, behavioral, and cognitive appraisal etiological models (Horowitz 1976, 1986; Janoff-Boulman, 1985; Keane, Fairbank, Caddell, Zimering, & Bender, 1985), the subjection to repeated trauma leads to the formation of PTSD. Within this conceptualization, those who develop PTSD will experience the traditional triad of core cluster symptoms (i.e., re-experiencing, avoidance, and hy-per-arousal). The formation of PTSD leads the victim to feeling trapped in the time of the trauma. For the victim, therefore, the trauma becomes the most significant occurrence of his or her life. This time distortion with the repeated re-experiencing phenomena leads to the reinforcement of mem-ory, which is formed in a distorted or impeded fashion. This, in turn, results in not only the formation of conscious memories about what occurred dur-ing and in the aftermath of the traumatic event(s), but also in the formation of automatic memory.

According to Bloom (1997), automatic memories include the auto-matic responses of dissociation and anger to trauma-related stimuli. Dissociation can lead to emotional numbing, while anger can lead to ag-gression and addictive behaviors. These latter behaviors can also be seen as part of the avoidance symptom cluster of PTSD. Subjection to repeated trauma, therefore, can generate a pattern of behaviour or cop-ing that allows one to survive and adapt to repeated threats. This adap-tive "over"-coping, however, becomes exaggerated and reinforced and can become maladaptive outside of the traumatic environment.

For example, a child may begin to daydream of a fantasised make-be-lieve world or environment in an attempt to imagine away abuse that is occurring. This tendency can lead to self-induced dissociation as a means of coping. When the trauma is over and the environment is normalised, however, such coping mechanisms can be very difficult to un-learn. The tendency to avoid reality through fantasizing is, therefore, at risk of becoming a learned coping mechanism in this example. Similarly, the child in this example may also respond to conscious memories of the abuse with fantasy-based avoidance. As this coping mechanism becomes paired with the re-experiencing phenomena of PTSD, the coping mechanism and symptoms may become increasingly difficult to unravel later on in therapy.

Depending on the developmental stage of the individual, these learned cognitions and behaviours could also influence the formation of personality, leading later to a propensity to enter situations that generate further feelings of learned helplessness (Herman, 1993). In such situations, one perceives any attempt to escape a trauma or negative outcome to be futile. In other words, no matter what the individual does to try to escape the trauma, the effect is believed to be the same in that there is no perceived escape. Relatively minor life events or stressors can generate feelings of learned helplessness once they have been established. Similarly, poor social support or social circumstances, including deprivation, can exacerbate such feelings in a traumatized individual. These later occurrences act as maintenance factors in relation to the learned coping styles used in later life. Learned helplessness, for example, can lead to the development of co-morbid diagnoses, such as depression and anxiety, which are commonly present with PTSD (Abramson, Seligman, & Teasdale, 1978; Maier & Seligman, 1976; Peterson & Seligman, 1983; Seligman, 1975).

Research has shown that the developmental or maturational stage of the individual at the time of traumatization is important in terms of etiology, symptom formation, and clinical presentation. Co-morbidity patterns, personality distortions, or partial or full arrest or regression of personality development may also be influenced by developmental stage. While more research is needed, some evidence in relation to this exists. For example, being traumatized after the age of 26 years is less likely to lead to a diagnosis of DESNOS and/or Complex PTSD, but not necessarily for a diagnosis of PTSD alone (van der Kolk, Mandel, Pelcovitz, & Roth, 1992). In addition, the formation of attachments and relationships, as well as subsequent social and occupational interactions, may be influenced by the stage of development at which traumatization occurs.

Van der Kolk (1996) and Roth, Newman, Pelcovitz, van der Kolk, and Mandel (1997), for example, found that those traumatized primarily in childhood are at greater risk for maladaptive functioning as they may not have had the chance to develop adaptive coping skills and personality structures. In such instances, the individuals may have never functioned normally before presenting for treatment. Such individuals are more likely to have spent years in psychiatric institutions or required psychiatric help (and form part of the numbers of the so called "revolving door patients") from outpatient agencies. Persons primarily subjected to multiple traumas in later childhood or adulthood, however, were more likely to have functioned relatively normally at some time in their lives.

Not all people subjected to repeated trauma in childhood or adulthood develop PTSD or DES, however. Some of those traumatized in childhood go on to develop other disorders, such as Borderline Personality Disorder (BPD) or Dissociative Identity Disorder (DID). It is postulated that those traumatized later in life do not go on to develop Complex PTSD, but may develop PTSD and enduring personality change following catastrophic stress (World Health Organization, 1992; F Code: 62.0). However, it is not known what differentiates those who develop Complex PTSD and a personality disorder or why other multiple trauma victims develop no psychiatric illness or personality distortion. Resiliency studies are lacking in this area of the stress disorders literature, although they have been described in relation to stress perception in general (Kobasa, 1979) and in the case of adults subjected to multiple traumas (e.g., combat veterans; Elder & Clipp, 1989).

Given Bloom's postulations and the outlined model of Complex PTSD highlighted above, it is clear that overlapping symptoms co-exist (e.g., the propensity to self-harm and changes in personality function). However, distinctions between the clinical characteristics of PTSD and BPD are documented in the literature. For example, those with BPD are more likely to be unable to tolerate being alone, whereas those with PTSD are more likely to be isolated (Gold, 1996; Gunderson, 1996; Gunderson & Sabo, 1993).

COPING AND LOCUS OF CONTROL

Exposure to trauma shifts locus of control from internality to externality and coping style from problem-solving-focused coping to emotion-focused coping. These mechanisms operate during the important periods of threat appraisal and during the relatively fluid symptoms of what DSM-IV terms as Acute Stress Disorder (Elder & Clipp, 1989; Perlin & Schooler, 1978). Even after PTSD has developed, locus of control and coping style have been postulated as crucial in relation to whether symptoms are perceived by the individual as being overwhelming or as simply being a burden to be "put up with" (Busuttil, 1995; Elder & Clipp, 1989). This point is, perhaps, easy to identify when the victim has been subjected to a single traumatic experience. The subjection to multiple traumas makes these concepts more difficult to envisage.

Use of the theoretical frameworks relating to the post-traumatic shift in coping style and locus of control are considered important in relation to the psycho-education material and cognitive restructuring methods employed in the rehabilitation of severely traumatized patients. However, it was felt that these theoretical frameworks did not adequately apply in this client group, and that the mechanisms governing coping and locus of control appear to be more complicated than the literature suggests. Further research would help to identify active mechanisms and help to improve therapeutic approaches (Busuttil, 1995).

STRUCTURED PROGRAMS AND REHABILITATION

The program described in this study comprised a rigidly structured treatment schedule that was incorporated within a therapeutic milieu setting. Structured programs have been used in military settings in the training of personnel who were poor recruit candidates (Novaco, 1977; Novaco, Cook, & Sarason, 1983). Recruits demonstrated a shift in locus of control (from externality to internality) and the promotion of personal characteristics and qualities, which improved function within a military environment. Structured programs were used in the management of PTSD in soldiers, for example, during the First World War (Hurst 1941; Lewis, 1919), post-Vietnam (Scurfield, 1993; Silver, 1986), post-Falklands War (O'Connell, 1991; cited in Hodgekinson & Steward, 1991), and after the Gulf War (Busuttil, Neal, Turnbull, Rollins, Blanche, & Herepath, 1995).

Other therapeutic principles incorporated into the program were therapeutic community approaches and milieu therapy (Bion, 1961; Clark, 1977). This means that patients have a say in their therapy and are listened to by the staff. They also take on some responsibilities for the running of the program and in choosing activities for their leisure time.

Incorporating these therapeutic principles and theoretical postulations, a 90-day program for the treatment of Complex PTSD was devised and is described below. The outcome over time of the first 25 participants is presented. Data collected by means of a psychometric assessment protocol utilized at the pre-treatment stage and at three follow-up periods was analyzed to see whether program attendance impacted symptoms and social and occupational functioning.

METHOD

Participants

This study is an open outcome report of the first consecutive 25 participants to date. They are currently at various stages of follow-up; therefore, not all participants have completed the one-year follow-up assessment. However, all participants have completed the program. Some patients were discharged over two years ago. To date, 18 patients have reached the one-year follow-up point and 12 have completed the one-year assessment. Of the six participants who did not participate in the one-year follow-up assessment, one was working abroad, two decided that they did not want any further contact with psychiatric services, and three participants could not be located.

The mean age at attendance was 26.2 years (range 17-45 years). Twenty-two participants were female and three were male. All were British Caucasian with the exception of one female of Afro-Caribbean origin. All gave a history of childhood sexual abuse and 23 were also victims of physical and emotional abuse. Ten participants also reported experiencing rape as an adult. At the time of treatment, two participants were divorced, four were engaged in long-term heterosexual relationships, and three were married. The remaining participants ($n = 16$) were single. Clinically, all participants met the DSM-IV diagnostic criteria for PTSD and the criteria for the diagnosis of Complex PTSD. All participants had received different 'working diagnoses' before entering the present study. Diagnoses included personality disorder ($n = 11$), schizophrenia ($n = 5$), severe depressive disorder ($n = 5$), bipolar affective disorder ($n = 1$), and dissociative disorder ($n = 3$).

Of the initial 25 patients, 21 had received treatment in a psychiatric hospital before admission to the unit. In 18 cases, in-patient management immediately preceded admission to the Complex PTSD program. In the other seven cases, treatment was preceded by outpatient support and supervision by a community mental health team. The 18 patients who were transferred to the Complex PTSD program directly from the hospital had been treated in the hospital continuously for a cumulative total of 27 years (mean = 25 months).

Participation was voluntary, and participants were not compensated for taking part in this study. Two subjects had been transferred to the program from other inpatient hospital settings and had been detained there under the 1983 Mental Health Act of England and Wales. These patients volunteered to enter the program despite being legally detained in hospital. They made sufficient progress during the program to be discharged from the hospital and from their mental health act detentions when the program was completed.

MEASURES

The psychometric assessment protocol included two measures of PTSD: the Clinician Administered PTSD Scale-1 (CAPS-1; Blake et al., 1990) and the Impact of Events Scale (IES; Horowitz, Wilner, & Alvarez, 1979). Two additional measures, the General Health Questionnaire-28 (GHQ-28; Goldberg & Hillier, 1979) and the Beck Depression Inventory (BDI; Beck, Rush, Shaw, & Emory, 1979) were included to assess co-morbidity.

The CAPS-1 symptom intensity score was derived by counting the intensity scores in the current symptom scale (Neal, Busuttil, Rollins, Herepath, Strike, & Turnbull, 1994). The CAPS-1 also gives a measure for occupational and social function on a five-point Likert scale. The CAPS-1 is a well-tested, structured interview schedule with excellent inter-rater reliability and validity (Wolfe & Keane, 1993). The IES (Horowitz et al., 1979) is a self-report fifteen-item scale that measures intrusive and avoidance phenomena of PTSD. This scale is commonly used as a screening tool for the presence of PTSD. It is scored on a four-point scale of 0, 1, 3, and 5. Subset scores for intrusion and avoidance are added to give a Total IES score. It has a high reliability and validity as a screening instrument for PTSD (McFall, Smith, & Roszell, 1990).

The GHQ-28 is a self-report scale that measures general psychiatric symptoms and gives a probability measure that the respondent will be a psychiatric case (cut-off = 5, maximum score possible = 28). The BDI is a self-report scale that assesses depressive symptoms. A score of 0-9 is minimal, 10-16 is mild, 17-29 is moderate, and 30-63 is severe.

PROCEDURES

Treatment comprised a highly structured residential program delivered to a closed group of participants for 90-days. Patients were admitted together on a pre-set admission date and the discharge date was set at the outset. The program was conducted from 9:00 am until 5:00 pm, five days a week, on a separate ward designated for the treatment of the selected participant population. The program was designed to take a maximum of six participants. The aims of the highly structured nature of this program are to promote a feeling of safety in the participants and to engender a predictable work routine, which allows specific space and time to disclose painful traumatic material. The setting of objectives within a definite time frame and a predetermined discharge date, known even before admission, is intended to aid motivation, to reduce avoidance of the issues that need to be confronted, and to aid discharge planning. The participants were expected to work hard and be discharged from the hospital at the end of the program. The program was designed to function as a tertiary referral service and currently operates in the private sector. Most of the patients admitted to the program were referred through mainstream (British) National Health Service (NHS) after having failed to respond to intervention available on the NHS.

Staff

Three therapists deliver therapy. Qualified psychiatric nursing staff and auxiliary nursing staff support them in this. The Consultant Psychiatrist retains ultimate clinical responsibility. All staff receive regular training in trauma theory and therapy. Staff work as an integrated team. Supervisory measures include time-tabled clinical supervision, secondary debriefing, and monitoring of patients by reading their daily diaries. Participants have weekly scheduled individual sessions with the consultant psychiatrist, allowing for progress and medication reviews. Staff and peer supervision, appropriate boundary setting, and maintenance are seen as essential to the smooth operation of the staff team.

Admission Criteria and Assessment

Assessment comprises a full outpatient psychiatric evaluation, including a mental status examination by a senior psychiatrist together with psychometric tests to confirm the presence of PTSD and co-morbid illness. A nursing assessment and therapist assessment follow. The assessment team then meets to discuss the particular needs of the patient and whether admission to the program is indicated. Patients must be motivated and willing to work. Actively violent patients are excluded, and self-harm must be under control. Dependence or heavy abuse of alcohol or illicit drugs is an exclusion criterion.

Therapeutic Techniques

The program is divided into three 30-day phases comprising: (a) Phase One: Interactive Psycho-education, Preparation for Disclosure, and Adjustment of Medication; (b) Phase Two: Disclosure of Traumatic Experiences; and (c) Phase Three: Cognitive Restructuring, Problem Solving, and Discharge Planning. It should be noted that phases one and three are carried out in a group format; whereas phase two is carried out on an individual basis. Several modules are focused upon during the initial phase of treatment. These modules include: (a) group work; (b) arousal reduction; (c) interactive psycho-education; (d) monitoring; and (e) medication.

Phase one. Group work is "closed" because group bonding is an important initial requirement since the program is run along therapeutic milieu lines (Clark, 1977); staff and patients, therefore, share responsibility ensuring that the program is run efficiently. The process begins initially by means of a trust exercise in which staff and patients participate. Group exercises identify participants' and staff aims, expectations, and goals. Ground rules and ward policies are also discussed. Boundary issues raised within the first few days of the program include the need for privacy, the rule that the staff share all knowledge of each patient, and that staff work as a cohesive team. Self-monitoring by use of a daily diary is introduced on the first day. The diaries are discussed further below.

Arousal reduction is delivered by means of ongoing didactic sessions and practical classes throughout the duration of the program. It includes relaxation exercises, anger management training, assertiveness training, role-play, and physical exercise.

Interactive psycho-education allows the development of insight and symptom management by the individual. A significant part of the first month is devoted to didactic sessions and discussion forums imparting theoretical knowledge. This allows the build up of some degree of psychological sophistication for each patient that is then used in Phase Two, the disclosure phase. Education helps the patients understand why it is important not to avoid the trauma and to confront and disclose in a controlled manner. Each topic is delivered in an interactive lecture format and then is discussed at length over a specifically designated discussion session. The main areas covered and explained thoroughly are: (a) the stress response; (b) PTSD; (c) Complex PTSD; (d) coping and locus of control; (e) relationships; (f) the meaning of psychological trauma; (g) empowerment; (h) illicit drug use; and (i) medications and their effects.

At the outset, participants are shown how to keep a daily diary in which they are encouraged to monitor their thoughts and feelings. They are encouraged to communicate concerns that they might otherwise be unable to raise during group sessions. Because staff read diaries on a daily basis, therapy may cover these areas without direct referral to the person who raised the index issue. Patients are also instructed to take notes on the didactic sessions, cognitive restructuring exercises, and lessons learned during the day. This allows them to take away a record of lessons after the program is complete, both for future reference and for use with the community psychiatric team after discharge. Daily review of the diaries by staff also allows therapy to cover all areas of the patients' ideas, concerns, and expectations, as well as monitoring progress. Material raised in the diaries is raised in discussion sessions, if pertinent, although the anonymity of the diaries is upheld at all times.

Patients are seen individually on a weekly basis by the senior psychiatrist in charge of their care. Patients also have access to a junior psychiatrist on a 24-hour basis. A weekly clinical meeting (ward round) allows staff team discussion of clinical management.

Patients are asked to complete an autobiography during this first phase. They are given a set of easy written guidelines to help them. This task is divided into three parts over three weeks. If writing about a particular part of the trauma is too difficult, they are to be brief. This allows therapists to see what can be disclosed easily and what is not as easy to disclose. It also helps to put the trauma into the context of the individual's life. Writing about trauma can be therapeutic in itself (Esterling, L'Abate, Murray, & Pennebaker, 1999).

The use of medication in the treatment of PTSD reflects current progress in relation to the biological etiological models of PTSD. Clinical experience in the management of complex PTSD patients has led to the use of the following combinations of medications: neuroleptics (for psychotic or pseudo-psychotic symptoms and dissociative experiences), antidepressants (primarily the SSRI's, for treating re-experiencing phenomena and hyperarousal of PTSD as well as co-morbid depression, obsessional thinking, and phobic and hypochondriacal symptoms), mood stabilizers (for reducing unpredictable, erratic mood swings), and/or clonidine (for increased arousal coupled with aggression and self-harming behavior). These classes of medications have all been noted in the literature in the treatment of PTSD (Friedman, 1988; Friedman, Southwick, & Charney, 1993; Kolb, Burris, & Griffiths,

1984; Wolf, Alavi, & Mosnaim, 1988; Yost, 1980). For more recent reviews of medication options, see Davidson and van der Kolk (1996), and Ratna and Barbenel (1997), or Friedman, Davidson, Mellman, and Southwick (2000).

Phase two. Processing and disclosures comprise the bulk of the second 30-day phase of treatment. The aim is to allow each patient to process the traumatic information, make connections with present belief systems and emotions, and to encourage them to move into the future. During the education phase, patients are taught that while the facts of what happened are important, what is just as important is what they did and how they coped with the trauma. Their memories of the traumas and how they perceive them in the present are also important. The sensory perceptions are also discussed and triggers are identified, so patients can feel equipped to deal with situations or triggers rather than avoid them. Issues concerning the meaning of the trauma are also discussed.

During this phase, actual disclosure is facilitated on an individual, rather than a group, basis. A therapist and nursing auxiliary conduct this disclosure. The therapist functions as the lead clinician for the session, delivering and directing the therapy, and the nurse acts as the patient's support. Peer supervision is delivered on a daily basis and psychotherapeutic supervision is delivered on at least a once-weekly basis. Patients usually disclose for up to six hours of therapeutic time per week, for a period of four weeks.

During disclosure, two main questions are asked by the therapist: What happened to you? and What did you feel about it? Patients discuss facts, feelings, sensory perceptions, and emotional reactions. These questions are in line with those asked during a classical critical incident stress debriefing (CISD) session (Busuttil & Busuttil, 1997; Dyregov, 1989; Mitchell, 1983, 1988, 1989; Mitchell & Derygov, 1993; Turnbull, 1992).

The emphasis is on learning and processing the traumatic material. Putting the theory learned during the psycho-education block into practice allows the development of insight into symptom formation and maintenance. This also allows the individual to process what has happened in the knowledge that avoidance has served to maintain the core cluster symptoms of PTSD. This aims to enhance motivation to confront what has happened. Patients are also able to make sense of what has happened and to vent their emotions, albeit in a socially acceptable way.

In group discussions, patients discuss common themes. Disclosure is not performed in a group format because some of the patients' disclosures might serve to traumatize other participants. The Disclosure phase begins by showing a video in which PTSD sufferers talk about their traumatic experiences and how they learned to cope (British Broadcasting Corporation, 1992). Patients depicted in the video are followed through their disclosure and at six weeks and six months following their attendance for similar 12-day "simple" PTSD rehabilitation program (Busuttil et al., 1995).

Phase three. Phase three of treatment consists of the following five modules: (a) cognitive restructuring and problem solving; (b) lines exercise; (c) ladder exercise; (d) life skills; and (e) discharge planning. Cognitive restructuring and problem solving techniques are used primarily in the Lines and Ladders exercises, originally described in the 12-day group rehabilitation program for the treatment of PTSD (Busuttil et al., 1995). Primary aims of these exercises are to promote self-awareness and personal responsibility so victims can attain and maintain an increased degree of control over their lives. The Lines exercise allows the trauma to be put into the perspective of one's life and identify positive and negative coping styles. These findings help the individual construct a multidimensional "ladder" with which the participant plans the future, and then presents the ladder to the group for reality testing.

The Lines exercise is assigned as a homework task, in which participants plot a time-graph of their lives. All significant high and low points and positive and negative events are plotted on the vertical axis (including a neutral midway point representing zero). The horizontal axis represents age in years. Patients include all major lifetime experiences, including the period when they were exposed to the traumatic stressor(s). They are also instructed to make diary notes of all the high and low points. This data enables them to make a presentation of their lives to the other group members in a graphical and coherent manner. Staff helps participants complete their homework if necessary.

Each Lines exercise is presented on a white board and is subjected to peer review and criticism. (While the presenter identifies the line graph point where traumatic events have occurred as a "traumatic episode," they never describe traumatic experiences in detail.) Two main therapeutic benefits emerge from the exercise. First, for the first time the patient puts the traumatic events into the perspective of the whole life experience. Comparing them with other high and low points gives a new perspective that permits the individual and the group to see that the stressors responsible for the Complex PTSD have become the dominant life experience. Second, the graph allows therapists to help the individual identify positive and negative coping patterns and behaviours prompted by the trauma and by other significant life events. These patterns and behaviours are noted in the individual's diary. Awareness of individuals' inherent coping styles is promoted. Maladaptive patterns are identified as maintaining factors of Complex PTSD. The effects of these negative patterns on other aspects of their lives (families, social contacts, etc.) are highlighted by group discussion.

The Ladder exercise naturally follows the Lines exercise. It permits the individual to plan the future by identifying short- and long-term goals, which are then presented to the entire group for discussion and reality testing. Plans must be as realistic as possible, keeping with the individual's coping styles as identified in the Lines exercise in order to plan for the future, with the emphasis placed on utilizing positive coping strategies and diminishing the use of maladaptive strategies. Group members draw a ladder with several rungs on a large sheet of paper. On the top rung, they place their long-term goal and on the bottom rung they place the lowest point in their lives. The individual then fills in the intervening rungs as steps to be taken to achieve the ultimate goal. The Ladders exercise is multidimensional, and includes as many relevant dimensions as are necessary for the individual (e.g., marital, family, social, occupational, and financial dimensions). Each individual presents his/her plans to the group in order to facilitate reality testing. The Ladder exercise is modified if need be and is then incorporated in the individual's diary for future reference and updating after discharge from the hospital. This exercise is thought to enhance powers of self-criticism, self-awareness, and self-esteem. The Ladders exercise also identifies other life skills required by the patient. For example, role-plays and social skills training are commonly needed and delivered. Each patient is given tailor made sessions as well as group sessions in assertiveness training, financial advice, and housing.

Liaison with each individual's National Health Service Community Mental Health Team (CMHT) starts before admission to the program. Two Care Program Approach Meetings (CPAs) are held during the program. The first takes place mid-way through the program, and the second approximately one week prior to discharge. The aim is to allow transfer of the patient to the NHS CMHT as smoothly as possible. Clinical responsibility is also transferred at discharge from the program. Liaison with other appropriate agencies is facilitated during this phase.

Follow-up at Six Weeks, Six Months, and One Year

Patients attend the hospital as a group together with their CMHT key mental health workers. Progress is reviewed by a therapist-led peer discussion, and by further reality testing of the goals set out in the original Ladders exercise. The senior psychiatrist conducts the individual assessment, and the psychometric assessment protocol is repeated. Advice is given, as required, to the CMHT. Telephone advice is also available to the CMHT, if required.

RESULTS

The data collected using the psychometric assessment protocol at the pre-treatment and three follow-up periods was analyzed to see whether attendance to the program made any difference to symptoms and social and occupational function. Outcome results over time, using parametric and non-parametric statistics (i.e., dependent t tests, and Wilcoxon signed rank tests), revealed that PTSD symptom status, depression symptom status, and function, as measured by the CAPS-1 occupational and social function subtests, significantly improved for all participants ($p < 0.05$) between pre-treatment and the six-week follow-up point. These improvements were generally maintained over time, as indicated by the one-year follow-up period scores. One exception was noted, however, where the comparison between the IES mean scores between pre-treatment and six months did not reach statistical significance ($p = 0.09$). No statistical differences were observed between all follow-up points ($p > 0.05$) (see Table 1). Interpretation of these findings, however, was limited by the fact that the number of subjects decreased over the follow-up period.

Table 2 summarizes the outcome for the subjects based on their co-morbid illness, behaviours, hospitalisations, and function. It must be noted, however, that there were several improvements that could not be measured using the psychometric tests employed by the study. These findings are also discussed below.

The Need for Continued Hospitalizations

After discharge from the program, participants were followed to assess for the need for continued care. Five participants required additional hospitalizations post-treatment. One patient has remained in a psychiatric hospital since discharge (approximately 18 months). This patient had been in hospital care continuously for a period of five years prior to admission to the program. A second patient spent a period of three months in the hospital following completion of the program because it was discovered she was of borderline IQ and required further rehabilitation using a simple behavioral program. The third participant spent six months in a psychiatric hospital following her discharge from the program due to the presence of suicidal ideations. Another patient was transferred to a short-term rehabilitation service where she spent six months hospitalized. The fifth patient was transferred to a long-term residential care facility. The other 20 participants spent a total of three months in a psychiatric hospital since discharge for a variety of minor crises. The 25 patients have, therefore, spent a total of three years in the hospital since their discharge from the treatment program. The 12 pa-

TABLE 2. Clinical Outcome Summary

Disturbance	Pre-treatment (*n* = 25)	Post-treatment to the nearest follow-up point. Cumulative follow-up period was 23 years 3 months.
Hospitalization for psychiatric problems	18 subjects transferred directly from hospital (Cumulative time in hospital prior to admission = 27 years)	(Hospitalization post-Tx) 1 subject = 1 yr 6 mos. 1 subject = 3 mos. (due to borderline intelligence) 2 subjects = 6 mos. (One is currently at College) 1 subject = transferred to long term residential care 20 subjects = cumulative total of 3 mos (range 1 day to 2 weeks)
Self-harm by cutting	18 subjects	5 subjects
History of Overdose	21 subjects history of over two overdoses in their past	3 overdoses in follow-up period
Jumping out of window in attempt at self-harm	None	1 incident
Eating disorder	Anorexia *n* = 3 Bulimia *n* = 2 Obesity *n* = 2	Anorexia *n* = 1 Bulimia *n* = 0 Obesity *n* = 1
Severe Agoraphobia Severe Obsessive Compulsive Disorder	1 subject 1 subject	Both cases much improved
Function Work/Education Mental Health Act Detention	None in employment or education immediately prior to admission 3 subjects detained under long term hospital orders at start of program	3 patients in college or further education; one manager of chain store 2 discharged from detention. 1 patient detained under a community detention order

tients who were discharged from the program over two years ago have not had any psychiatric admissions lasting over a few days since that time.

Self-Harming Behaviors

Prior to treatment, three-quarters of the participants reported repeatedly engaging in self-harming behaviors. In particular, the following behaviors were reported: (a) cutting; (b) bashing of the head; (c) genital mutilation; (d) repeated use of ligatures; and (e) repeated overdoses. A significant reduction was found in the frequency of such behaviors for all participants at six-months post-treatment, with only five participants reporting any continuation of self-harming behaviors. Three overdose attempts did occur post-treatment, but participants sought help immediately in all three cases. One other attempt at self-harm was reported and involved the participant jumping out of a second floor window. This behavior led to a hospital admission for that participant.

Eating Disorders

Seven patients were suffering from an eating disorder prior to treatment, including anorexia nervosa ($n = 3$), bulimia ($n = 2$), or obesity ($n = 2$). Following treatment, one patient continued to suffer from anorexia and another remained severely obese. The other four participants, however, did not continue to display features of an eating disorder.

Agoraphobia

One patient suffered from severe agoraphobia along with PTSD and depression. This patient's agoraphobia improved and, at one-year follow-up, she could go out of her house alone. By two years, she had visited another continent with her husband and had been able to face having extensive gynecological operations. She could not have entertained the thought of obtaining a physical examination prior to entering the program.

Obsessive-Compulsive Disorder

One patient suffered severe symptoms of obsessive-compulsive disorder. In this case, while obsessive thinking remained present at one year follow-up, ritual behaviors had diminished dramatically, allowing some return of function, including attendance of a college course.

Functional Improvements

All but two participants improved from a functional point of view. For example, three patients began attending college and a fourth was promoted to a managerial position in a chain store. Prior to admission to the program, these four patients had been in a psychiatric hospital for a total of five years.

The Mental Health Act Status

On admission to the program, three patients were detained in the hospital under Section 3 of the England and Wales' Mental Health Act (1983) for over six months (range 1-3 years). By the time of discharge from the hospital, two patients were successfully removed from their Section and the other had her Section transferred to a community supervision section (Section 117, Mental Health Act, 1983).

DISCUSSION

While evaluation of this program is at an early stage, the initial findings are clearly encouraging. The population treated in this program was severely ill and most had been chronically hospitalized prior to their participation. Motivation and the quality of follow-up psychiatric care in the community are important factors in keeping these patients out of the hospital for the long-term. The second phase of the program, disclosure, appears to be the most therapeutic, in that the patients report improved affect after they have told their stories. However, this would not be possible without the safety of an inpatient unit and the preparation they receive before and during the psycho-education phase, as it is probable that without the knowledge given during this phase the patient would continue to avoid talking about the traumatic experience.

Adjustment in the medications as described also makes a large difference in the mental states in many of the patients treated thus far. Furthermore, the final phase of cognitive restructuring, problem solving, and discharge planning was found to represent a key factor in being rehabilitated back into the community. While the results of the present study seem to indicate that the treatment program represents a valid

means of treating PTSD in an inpatient group setting, certain components of the treatment protocol (i.e., interactive psycho-education and
cognitive behavior therapy) have also been used in other outpatient
treatment programs for PTSD with good results at six-month follow-up
assessments (Lubin, Loris, Burt, Johnson, 1998), although controlled
studies are lacking. Future studies may want to investigate the validity
of the proposed treatment program, therefore, in controlled, outpatient
settings.

The debate regarding a trauma-focused approach versus a rehabilitation approach as the best option for use in multiply traumatized veterans
and those who are chronically unwell is highlighted in the literature
(Johnson, 1997; Johnson & Lubin, 1997). This debate has highlighted
that exposure to the trauma by means of talking about it or undergoing
exposure therapy to it may not be as helpful as previously thought and
that a rehabilitation approach to treatment may be the best treatment
method for severely ill chronic PTSD sufferers. The program presented
here with indications of improved symptomatology and function suggests that a combination of the two approaches worked with the sample
of multiple trauma victims in this study. Further research may clarify
the position.

There has also been some debate in the literature as to whether inpatient programs run by staff on wards that are dedicated to the treatment of
PTSD are worthwhile. Some studies investigating the benefits of such a
setting have reported good outcomes, especially if the intervention is implemented shortly following traumatization, as was the case in a 12-day
residential brief group therapy rehabilitation program devised for the military (Busuttil et al., 1995). Other inpatient programs, however, have not
proven to be as helpful. For example, some inpatient programs dedicated
to the treatment of chronic PTSD in American Vietnam veterans have not
been very successful in reducing PTSD symptomology or post-treatment
functioning in (Rosenheck, Fontana, & Errera, 1997). The findings of this
90-day program contradict these findings although further evaluation is
required. Some workers have suggested that one of the reasons as to why
some veteran's programs fail is because many participants were exposed
to several lifetime traumas before Vietnam (Shalev, 1997). Busuttil et al.
(1995) formed the same impression after treating British veterans with a
short 12-day program. The 90-day program was specifically designed to
cater to these victims of multiple traumas, however.

Creamer, Morris, Biddle, and Elliott (1999) assessed the outcomes of a
large cohort ($n = 419$) Australian Vietnam veterans who completed a
12-week hospital-based program. Significant improvements at three- and

nine-month's follow-up were demonstrated. The findings suggest that the treatment of PTSD may benefit from the use of inpatient group programs. Initial results from the present study seem to provide further support for this notion.

There are several limitations to the present study, including a small sample size and the uncontrolled design of the study. In addition, there are other areas that require evaluation but that were not assessed here. For example, which aspects of this multimodal program are most efficacious? Another facet would be to study the effects of the program in relation to shift in locus of control and coping style pre and post treatment. To date, no research has been conducted on the impact of multiple traumas versus a singular trauma on these mechanisms. Similarly, developmental stage at the time of traumatization has not yet been studied for its effects on later locus of control or coping style.

Full assessment of the program presented here will require further work. Ideally, future investigations will be conducted using controlled multi-centre studies. However, the program shows promise in this needy chronically ill population of psychiatric patients.

REFERENCES

Abramson, L. Y., Seligman, M. E., & Teasdale, J. D. (1978). Learned helplessness in humans: Critique and reformulation. *Journal of Abnormal Psychology, 87,* 49-74.

American Psychiatric Association. (1994). *Diagnostic and statistical manual of mental disorders* (4th ed.). Washington, DC: Author.

Beck, A. T., Rush, A., Shaw, B. F., & Emory, G. (1979). *Cognitive therapy of depression.* New York: Guilford Press.

Bion, W. R. (1961). *Experiences in groups.* London: Tavistock.

Blake, D., Weathers, F., Nagy, L., Kaloupek, D. G., Klaminzer, G., Charney, D. S., & Keane, T. M. (1990). A clinician rating scale for assessing current and lifetime PTSD: The CAPS-1. *The Behaviour Therapist, 13,* 187-188.

Bloom, S. (1997). *Creating sanctuary. Toward the evolution of sane societies.* London: Routledge.

British Broadcasting Corporation. (1992). *Within walls* [Motion picture]. (Available from the British Broadcasting Corporation, Bush House, Bush Strand London, England WC2R 2ES.)

Burgess, A., & Holmstrom, L. (1976). Coping behavior of the rape victim. *American Journal of Psychiatry, 131,* 981-985.

Burgess, A., & Holmstrom, L. (1979). Adaptive strategies and recovery from rape. *American Journal of Psychiatry, 136,* 1278-1282.

Burgess, A., Holmstrom, L., Marmar, C. & Krupnick, J. (1980). Pathological grief and the activation of latent self-images. *American Journal of Psychiatry, 137,* 1137-1162.

Busuttil, W. (1993). Separation: The effects on service families. *Defence Medical Services Military Psychiatry Conference. Royal Army Medical College.* London: Millbank.

Busuttil, W. (1995). *Interventions in post traumatic stress syndromes: Implications for military and emergency service organisations.* Unpublished master's thesis, University of London, London, England.

Busuttil, W. (2000, March). *Group programmes.* In *Group approaches in the treatment of simple and complex PTSD in victims of incarceration: Approaches used in recent release of Australian care workers.* Symposium conducted at the World Conference of the International Society for Traumatic Stress Studies, Melbourne, Australia.

Busuttil, W., Aquilina, C., & Busuttil, A. M. C. (1993). Early life trauma, infertility and late Life paranoia: A relationship with post traumatic stress disorder? *International Journal of Geriatric Psychiatry, 8,* 693-695.

Busuttil, W., & Busuttil, A. M. C. (1997). Debriefing and crisis intervention. In D. Black, M. Newman, J. Harris Hendriks, & G. Mezey (Eds.), *Psychological trauma: A developmental approach* (pp. 238-249). London: Gaskell.

Busuttil, W., Neal, L. A., Turnbull, G. J., Rollins, J., Blanche, N., & Herepath, R. (1995). Incorporating psychological debriefing techniques within a brief group psychotherapy programme for the treatment of post-traumatic stress disorder. *British Journal of Psychiatry, 152,* 164-173.

Chodoff, P. (1963). The late effects of the concentration camp syndrome. *Archives of General Psychiatry, 8,* 323-333.

Clark, D. H. (1977). The therapeutic community. *British Journal of Psychiatry, 131,* 553-564.

Creamer, M., Morris, P., Biddle, D., & Elliott, P. (1999). Treatment outcome in Australian veterans with combat related posttraumatic stress disorder: A cause for cautious optimism? *Journal of Traumatic Stress, 12,* 625-641.

Davidson, J. R. T., & van der Kolk, B. A. (1996). The psychopharmacological treatment of post traumatic stress disorder. In B. A. van der Kolk, A. C. McFarlane, & L. Weisaeth (Eds.), *Traumatic stress: The effects of overwhelming experience on mind, body, and society* (pp. 510-524). New York: Guilford Press.

Dyregov, A. (1989). Caring for helpers in disaster situations: Psychological debriefing. *Disaster Management, 2,* 25-30.

Eitinger, L. (1959). The incidence of mental disease among refugees in Norway. *The Journal of Mental Science, 105,* 326-338.

Eitinger, L. (1961). Pathology of the concentration camp syndrome. *Archives of General Psychiatry, 5,* 371-379.

Eitinger, L. (1964). *Concentration camp survivors in Norway and Israel.* Oslo, Norway: Oslo University Press.

Elder, G. H., & Clipp, E. C. (1989). Combat experience and emotional health: Impairment and resilience in later life. *Journal of Personality, 57,* 311-341.

Esterling, B. A., L'Abate, L., Murray, E. J., & Pennebaker, J. W. (1999). Empirical foundations for writing in prevention and psychotherapy: Mental and physical health outcomes. *Clinical Psychology Review, 19*(1), 79-96.

Friedman, M. J. (1988). Toward rational pharmacotherapy for post traumatic stress disorder: An interim report. *American Journal of Psychiatry, 143,* 281-285.

Friedman, M. J., Southwick, S. M., & Charney, D. S. (1993). Pharmacotherapy for recently evacuated military casualties. *Military Medicine, 158*, 493-497.

Friedman, M. J., Davidson, J. R. T., Mellman, T. A., & Southwick, S. M. (2000). Pharmacotherapy. In E. B. Foa, T. M. Keane, & M. J. Friedman (Eds.), *Effective treatments for PTSD: Practice guidelines from the International Society for Traumatic Stress Studies* (pp. 84-105). New York: Guilford Press.

Gold, J. (1996). The intolerance of aloneness. *American Journal of Psychiatry, 153*, 749-750.

Goldberg, D. P., & Hillier, V. F. (1979). A scaled version of the General Health Questionnaire. *Psychological Medicine, 9*, 139-145.

Gunderson, J. (1996). The borderline patient's intolerance of aloneness: Insecure attachments and therapist availability. *American Journal of Psychiatry, 153*, 752-758.

Gunderson, J., & Sabo, A. N. (1993). The phenomenologial and conceptual interface between Borderline Personality Disorder and PTSD. *American Journal of Psychiatry, 150*, 19-27.

Herman, J. L. (1992). Complex PTSD: A syndrome in survivors of prolonged and repeated trauma. *Journal of Traumatic Stress, 5*, 377-391.

Herman, J. L. (1993). Sequelae of prolonged and repeated trauma: Evidence for a complex post traumatic stress syndrome (DESNOS). In J. R. T. Davidson & E. B. Foa (Eds.), *Post traumatic stress disorder. DSM-IV and beyond* (pp. 213-228). Washington DC: American Psychiatric Press.

Hodgekinson, P. E., & Steward, M. (Eds.) (1991). *Coping with catastrophe: A handbook of disaster management.* London: Routledge.

Horowitz, M. J. (1976). *Stress response syndromes.* New York: Jason Aronson.

Horowitz, M. J. (1986). *Stress response syndromes* (2nd ed.). New York: Jason Aronson.

Horowitz, M. J., Wilner, N., & Alvarez, W. (1979). Impact of events scale: A measure of subjective stress. *Psychosomatic Medicine, 41*, 209-218.

Hurst, A. (1941). *Medical diseases of war.* London: Edward Arnold.

Janoff-Bulman, R. (1985). The aftermath of victimisation: Rebuilding shattered assumptions. In C. R. Figley (Ed.), *Trauma and its wake: The study and treatment of post traumatic stress disorder* (Vol. 1 pp. 15-35). New York: Brunner Mazel.

Johnson, D. R. (1997). Introduction: Inside the specialized inpatient PTSD units of the department of veterans affairs. *Journal of Traumatic Stress, 10*, 357-360.

Johnson, D. R., & Lubin, H. (1997). Treatment preferences of Vietnam veterans with post traumatic stress disorder. *Journal of Traumatic Stress, 10*, 391-405.

Keane, T. M., Fairbank, J. A., Caddell, R. T., Zimering, R. T., & Bender, M. E. (1985). A behavioural approach to assessing and treating PTSD in Vietnam veterans. In C. R. Figley (Ed.), *Trauma and its wake: The study and treatment of post traumatic stress disorder* (Vol. 1, pp. 257-294). New York: Brunner Mazel.

Kilpatrick, D. G., Saunders, B. E., & Vernonen, L. J. (1987). Criminal victimisation: Lifetime prevalence, reporting to police, and psychological impact. *Crime and Delinquency, 33*, 479-489.

Kobasa, S. C. (1979). Stressful life events, personality, and health: An inquiry into hardiness. *Journal of Personality and Social Psychology, 37*, 1-11.

Kolb, L. C., Burris, B. C., & Griffiths, S. (1984). Propranolol and clonidine in treatment of chronic post-traumatic stress disorders of war. In B. A. van der Kolk (Ed.), *Post-traumatic stress disorder: Psychological and biological sequelae* (pp. 97-105). Washington DC: American Psychiatric Press.

Lewis, T. (1917). *Report upon soldiers returned as cases of "Disordered Action of the Heart" (DAH) or "Vulvular Disease of the Heart" (VDH)*. Medical Research Committee. London: Longmans, Green & Co.

Lubin, H., Loris, M., Burt, J., & Johnson, D. R. (1998). Efficacy of psychoeducational group therapy in reducing the symptoms of post traumatic stress disorder among multiply traumatised women. *American Journal of Psychiatry, 155*, 1172-1177.

Maier, S. F., & Seligman, M. E. (1976). Learned helplessness: Theory and evidence. *Journal of Experimental Psychology: General, 105*, 3-46.

McFall, M. E., Smith, D. E., & Roszell, D. K. (1990). Convergent validity of measures of PTSD in Vietnam Combat veterans. *American Journal of Psychiatry, 147*, 645-648.

Mental Health Act. (1983). Information available from http://www.doh.gov.uk/mhact1983/index.htm

Mitchell, J. T. (1983). When disaster strikes. The critical incident stress debriefing process. *Journal of Emergency Medical Services, 8*, 36-39.

Mitchell, J. T. (1988). The history and status and future of critical incident stress debriefings. *Journal of Emergency Medical Services, November*, 47-52.

Mitchell, J. T. (1989). Development and functions of a critical incident stress debriefing team. *Journal of Emergency Medical Services, December*, 43-46.

Mitchell, J. T., & Dyregrov, A. (1993). Traumatic stress in disaster workers and emergency personnel. Prevention and intervention. In J. P. Wilson & B. Raphael (Eds.), *International handbook of traumatic stress syndromes* (pp. 905-914). New York: Plenum Press.

Neal, L. A., Busuttil, W., Rollins, J., Herepath, R., Strike, P., & Turnbull, G. (1994). Convergent validity of measures of post-traumatic stress disorder in a mixed military and civilian population. *Journal of Traumatic Stress, 7*, 447-455.

Novaco, R. (1977). A stress inoculation approach to anger management in the training of law enforcement officers. *American Journal of Community Psychology, 5*, 327-346.

Novaco, R., Cook, T. M., & Sarason, I. G. (1983). Military recruit training. An arena for stress-coping skills. In D. Meichenbaum & M. E. Jaremko (Eds.), *Stress reduction and prevention* (pp. 377-417). New York: Plenum Press.

Perlin, H. J., & Schooler, C. (1978). The structure of coping. *Journal of Health and Social Behaviour, 19*, 433-448.

Peterson, C., & Seligman, M. E. P. (1983). Learned helplessness and victimisation. *Journal of Social Issues, 39*, 105-118.

Psychiatric Division of the Royal Air Force Medical Service. (1993). The management of hostages after release. *Psychiatric Bulletin of the Royal College of Psychiatrists, 17*, 35-37.

Ratna, L., & Barbenel, D. (1997). Pharmacotherapy of PTSD. *International Journal of Psychiatry in Clinical Practice, 1*, 169-177.

Rosenheck, R., Fontana, A., & Errera, P. (1997). Inpatient treatment of war related posttraumatic stress disorder: A 20 year perspective. *Journal of Traumatic Stress, 10,* 407-415.

Roth, S., Newman, E., Pelcovitz, D., van der Kolk, B. A., & Mandel, F. (1997). Complex PTSD in victims exposed to sexual and physical abuse: Results from the DSM-IV field trial for posttraumatic stress disorder. *Journal of Traumatic Stress, 10,* 539-556.

Scurfield, R. M. (1993). Treatment of post traumatic stress disorder among Vietnam veterans. In J. P. Wilson & B. Raphael (Eds.), *International handbook of traumatic stress syndromes* (pp. 879-888). New York: Plenum Press.

Seligman, M. E. P. (1975). *Helplessness: On depression, development, and death.* San Francisco: Freeman.

Shalev, A. Y. (1997). Treatment of prolonged post traumatic stress disorder–learning from experience. *Journal of Traumatic Stress, 10,* 415-423.

Silver, S. M. (1986). An inpatient programme for PTSD. Context as treatment. In C. R. Figley (Ed.), *Trauma and its wake* (Vol. 2, pp. 213-231). New York: Brunner Mazel.

Thygesen, P., Hermann, K., & Willanger, R. (1970). Concentration camp survivors in Denmark: Persecution, disease, compensation. *Danish Medical Bulletin, 17,* 65-108.

Turnbull, G. J. (1992). Debriefing British POWs after the Gulf War and released hostages from Lebanon. *WISMIC (World wide Veterans Foundation International Socio-Medical Information Centre) Newsletter, 4*(1), 4-6.

Turnbull, G. J., & Busuttil W. (1992a, September). *The de-briefing of British Gulf prisoners of war and Beirut hostages.* Symposium conducted at the World Conference of the International Society for Traumatic Stress Studies, Amsterdam, The Netherlands.

Turnbull, G. J., & Busuttil W. (1992b, September). *Hostage de-briefing.* Symposium conducted at the World Conference of the International Society for Traumatic Stress Studies, Amsterdam, The Netherlands.

Turner, S., & Gorst-Unsworth, C. (1990). Psychological sequelae of torture: A descriptive model. *British Journal of Psychiatry, 157,* 475-480.

van der Kolk, B. A. (1996). Trauma and memory. In B. A. van der Kolk, A. McFarlane, & L.Weisaeth (Eds.), *Traumatic stress* (pp. 279-302). New York: Guilford.

van der Kolk, B. A., Mandel, F., Pelcovitz, D., & Roth. S. (1992, September). *Update of DESNOS data analysis.* Presentation at the World Conference of the International Society for Traumatic Stress Studies, Amsterdam, The Netherlands.

van der Kolk, B. A., Roth. S., Pelcovitz, D., & Mandel, F. (1994). *Complex Post traumatic stress disorder. Results from the DSM-IV Field trial for PTSD.* New York: American Psychiatric Association.

Wolf, M. E., Alavi, A., & Mosnaim, A. D. (1988). Posttraumatic stress disorder in Vietnam veterans: Clinical and EEG findings: Possible therapeutic effects of carbamazepine. *Biological Psychiatry, 23,* 642-644.

Wolfe, J., & Keane, T. M. (1993). New perspectives in the assessment and diagnosis of combat-related post traumatic stress disorder. In J. P. Wilson & B. Raphael (Eds.), *International handbook of traumatic stress syndromes* (pp. 165-177). New York: Plenum.

World Health Organization. (1992). *International statistical classification of disease and related health problems* (10th ed.). Geneva: Author.

Yost, J. (1980). The psychopharmachologic treatment of the delayed stress syndrome in Vietnam veterans. In T. Williams (Ed.), *Post-traumatic stress disorders of the Vietnam veteran* (pp. 124-130). Columbus, OH: Disabled American Veterans.

How Schools Respond
to Traumatic Events:
Debriefing Interventions and Beyond

Mary Beth Williams

SUMMARY. School systems face crises of a variety of types and forms, including the suicide death of a student, the death of a teacher, mass shootings, and the aftermath of terrorist attacks. This article examines ways for school systems to deal with the aftermath of those crises, both immediately and in the long term. Suggestions for classroom interventions, group experiences, and homework assignments are included. The impact of terrorism on school personnel is also discussed. *[Article copies available for a fee from The Haworth Document Delivery Service: 1-800-HAWORTH. E-mail address: <docdelivery@haworthpress.com> Website: <http://www.HaworthPress.com> © 2006 by The Haworth Press, Inc. All rights reserved.]*

KEYWORDS. Terrorism, schools, crisis, debriefing, defusing, classroom interventions

---

Address correspondence to Dr. Mary Beth Williams, 9 North Third Street, # 14, Warrenton, VA 20186 (E-mail: mbethwms@infionline.net).

The author would like to acknowledge the entire staff of the Falls Church City Public Schools for the dedication to the lives of the children of Falls Church City that they give.

[Haworth co-indexing entry note]: "How Schools Respond to Traumatic Events: Debriefing Interventions and Beyond." Williams, Mary Beth. Co-published simultaneously in *Journal of Aggression, Maltreatment & Trauma* (The Haworth Maltreatment & Trauma Press, an imprint of The Haworth Press, Inc.) Vol. 12, No. 1/2, 2006, pp. 57-81; and: *Trauma Treatment Techniques: Innovative Trends* (ed: Jacqueline Garrick, and Mary Beth Williams) The Haworth Maltreatment & Trauma Press, an imprint of The Haworth Press, Inc., 2006, pp. 57-81. Single or multiple copies of this article are available for a fee from The Haworth Document Delivery Service [1-800-HAWORTH, 9:00 a.m. - 5:00 p.m. (EST). E-mail address: docdelivery@haworthpress.com].

doi:10.1300/J146v12n01_04

On September 11, 2001, terrorists attacked both the World Trade Center in New York City and the Pentagon in Washington, DC. The impact of this attack was felt across the United States, as the media's coverage provided viewers with repeated exposure to the destruction that occurred in its wake. Even in school buildings, teachers and other staff members had difficulty looking away from the broadcasts of the attacks and returning to their classroom duties. These events, and subsequent events related to the two snipers who terrorized the Washington, DC-Richmond (VA) corridor, caused residents of this area to question the safety and predictability of their world. This author was the school social worker for Falls Church City Public Schools, a small school system located in Virginia only a few minutes from downtown Washington, DC. The position of school social worker provided the author with a unique opportunity to examine school responses to these events, as well as the efficacy of those responses. This article explores those responses to the September 11th terrorist attack, and then gives recommendations for the development of a protocol for schools' response.

RESPONSE TO THE SEPTEMBER 11TH ATTACKS: WHEN LITTLE WAS ENOUGH

A major source of immediate concern for all of the metropolitan school systems in the Washington, DC area was how to assist those children who had a parent or other significant person among the casualties cope with their loss. A meeting with all of the after school daycare providers was, therefore, immediately held in the central office to discuss the possible reactions of these children. The school student service team members (i.e., psychologists and school social worker) focused on how to relate to potentially traumatized children during this initial meeting. Since school personnel did not know if any student or staff member had experienced the death or injury of a loved one at that time, the system did not mobilize the crisis response team to immediately intervene in the schools. In fact, the decision was made to maintain the students' regular routine until more information could be accumulated. In this case, to avoid promoting hysteria with the premature presence of a crisis team it was decided that initially "doing less was more than enough" to maintain an attitude of calmness and support.

Parents who were seriously impacted by the attack, either directly or through their own personal fears and vulnerabilities, began to retrieve their children from school, despite the staff's belief that it would have been better for the children to remain in a routine environment. Upon learning that one father had taken all three of his children from school, this author made a home visit to check on the family. Upon arrival at the home, this author saw that the father was frantically throwing things in the back of his car. He was planning to leave the area as soon as possible for a cabin in North Carolina so that "his children would not have to smell the smoke from the City burning." His wife was standing by in utter amazement, unable to stop her husband's frantic behavior. To no avail, the author tried to calm him down and show him that his behavior was scaring both his wife and children. He emphatically told the author to leave and then got in the car and sped down the highway.

This parent was unable to see that he was modeling an ineffective means of dealing with stress for his children. It is very likely that his panicked behaviors conveyed his terror and compromised sense of trust and safety to his children. In addition, his dismissal of my attempts to discuss the situation conveyed to the children that the school social worker was also no longer a safe person to trust or rely on for reliable guidance in a crisis situation. The family returned about five days later when "the world did not end." Following their return, the children demonstrated an increasing number of problems, including overeating, migraines, and sleep disturbances. Similarly, his wife has reportedly experienced post-traumatic stress reactions to this and other subsequent crises.

The Falls Church City Public Schools were fortunate in that none of their students had directly lost a loved one in the September 11th terrorist attacks. However, both the school system and the Falls Church City government implemented measures to safeguard the welfare of students and staff and to assist them in coping with potential losses of or injuries to family members. On September 20, 2001, superintendent Mary Ellen Shaw wrote in the *Falls Church News Press*:

> We feared our students and staff members could have family members injured or killed . . . we prepared to take care of students whose parents were not able to get home at their normal time (beyond the normal closing time). Teachers volunteered to stay beyond the normal hours and bus drivers were alerted to return students to school if parents were not home as planned. The staff of the day care programs came in an hour early to meet with the school psychologists and social worker to discuss how to answer students' questions and to support students if they were upset. (p. 2)

In addition, the metropolitan area school superintendents decided, as a group, to close all schools and cancel all school activities for the day following the attacks in an attempt to guard against additional attacks. This decision was also made so that police, fire, and rescue services could focus their attention on assisting rescue efforts at the Pentagon.

The schools re-opened on September 13, 2001, two days after the attacks. Staff members were on alert for those students who were in need of debriefing, defusing, or one-on-one interventions. According to staff reports, however, very few interventions were actually needed. In fact, students appeared to return to the task at hand (i.e., academic instruction and performance) without a great deal of disruption. It may have been that the students were glad to return to the safety of the school setting. In fact, the routine of school may have been a pleasurable contrast to the sudden chaos and insecurity of their world at large.

School announcements were also used to acknowledge the events of the preceding 48 hours, and to pull the student body together in the sudden atmosphere of cultural suspicion and blame. For example, George Mason High School and Middle School opened on September 13 with the following announcement:

> Good morning, Mustangs. We are glad to have our school community back together today . . . the immediate victims of these tragedies in New York, Pennsylvania, and here in Virginia were people of all ages, all colors, and all beliefs. These unfortunate souls number in the thousands. Those of us who grieve over these attacks and feel sad and angry about them are many, many millions . . . We speak many languages, we hold many different religious beliefs and we often dress and look different from one another. But we are united in that we are all, in a very real sense, victims of what happened on Tuesday.
>
> We have already begun to hear reports on the news that certain individuals may be responsible for these acts of terrorism . . . Let us hope that everyone in the world is capable of understanding that, whoever the responsible parties turn out to be, they most certainly do not represent an entire group of people with whom they might share a culture, a heritage, a language or a religion. The person sitting next to you or me might look and be different from you or me in many ways, but that doesn't mean that he or she is any less pained by all of this than are you or I. I am sure that we all feel hurt by what has happened and that each of us feels that hurt in our own private way. George Mason is a wonderfully diverse school community . . . It is to be celebrated that we all have come to be in the

same school together. In this time of national and international tragedy and mourning, let's count on each other's support and understanding to move forward together. The flags outside our building fly at half-mast this morning to honor the victims and heroic rescue workers who perished on Tuesday. This morning's minute of silence will be extended to honor their memory as well.

TERRORISM AS A SPECIAL TYPE OF CRISIS

In a presentation at the annual meeting of the American Psychological Association (APA), Diane Myers (2001) noted, "terrorism intends, as its primary goal, to terrify, to overpower with intense fear, to intimidate to achieve an end." She further stated, "terrorists use their abilities to psychologically injure, manipulate, and control the behavior of individuals and populations." They generally strike without warning to produce maximum amounts of social and psychological disruption. Terrorist attacks abruptly change the realities of everyday lives and represent serious threats to the safety and security of the victimized population. The scope of actual physical destruction from these attacks is generally great in intensity, leading to greater psychological impact than a traumatic event that does not lead to such chaos (Myers, 2001). Often, these events result in gruesome, grotesque situations that make recovery efforts a particularly horrific experience. Even where there is only one victim, the intense law enforcement response and crime scene investigation is often exposed to television cameras from all over the world, bringing anguish and repeated stress to all who watch the news coverage, regardless of their relationships with the deceased.

These attacks were intentional, purposely inflicting pain and despair. After September 11th, the worlds of many children in the United States were no longer benign and predictable. According to Myers (2001), the attacks sent the following message: "We can get you anywhere, at any time. If we are willing to kill your children, we will not hesitate to kill you. There is no one who can protect you."

The consequences of a terrorist attack therefore include psychological as well as physical casualties. As Bloom (2001) stated in a message to the International Society of Traumatic Stress Studies, "Our memories literally engrave vivid nonverbal imprints of the sounds, the sights, the body sensations and emotions that haunt us long into the future, triggered by even faint reminders of the terrible pain of mass destruction. Today, we are a traumatized nation, impaired by the overwhelming nature of unimaginable events . . . Emotional safety can only be restored by giving ourselves time to grieve for our losses, to find meaning in what happened, and, most important of all, to find ways to rebuild a shattered trust." Similar statements could apply to the round-the-clock images on CNN of the Ponderosa Restaurant in Ashland, Virginia, the Home Depot parking lot in Falls Church, Virginia, or the other locations that flooded the television screen during the snipers' reign of terror during the fall of 2002.

RESPONDING TO TERRORIST ATTACKS: THE COMMUNITY LEVEL

According to Everly and Mitchell (2001), community leaders may want to consider eight factors when developing community-level response and intervention plans in the event of terrorist attacks. First, crisis intervention hot lines and walk-in crisis intervention facilities should be available to help citizens cope with the ramifications of the terrorist activities. Second, emergency response personnel ideally need pre-incident training, as well as ongoing psychological support to cope with their own response to a terrorist attack and the secondary traumatization that may result from helping others.

Third, Everly and Mitchell recommend that it is essential to provide credible information to all members of the targeted community to reduce the sense of psychological uncertainty and loss of control that often accompanies a terrorist attack. This information can be dispensed via the mass media and more personal communications (e.g., those from school officials to the parents) to contradict the sense of chaos and subsequent rumors that often follow a terrorist attack. Furthermore, police need to provide information openly, even if doing so might initially cause the recipient(s) more fear. To accomplish this task, however, the police need to be able to disclose the relevant information without threat of suit or without repeated bombardment of reporters asking team leaders to disclose confidential case-related information.

Everly and Mitchell's fourth recommendation is to try to re-establish a sense of physical safety for the public to disarm the intended impact of a terrorist attack, with special considerations for children, the elderly, and the infirm. For example, placing uniformed law enforcement officers in cruisers near schools can be reassuring once the purpose of their presence has been properly explained to the students and their parents. Fifth, the ability to enlist the help of local political, educational, medical, economic, and religious leaders is recommended to facilitate communications, calm fears, provide personal crisis intervention, and instill hope. Inter-denominational religious services can be used to bring solace and calm fears, further enabling the community to heal following a terrorist attack. A sixth recommended response to terrorism involves re-establishing normal communication, transportation, school, and work schedules as soon as possible to foster the sense of control and predictability that existed prior to the attack. While routines remain disrupted, the level of stress one feels is likely to continue. Similarly, trying to maintain a normal routine, with a healthy respect for hypervigilance and attentiveness to one's surroundings, is important. Although parents cannot and should not reassure their children of ultimate safety when such safety is a myth, maintaining close to normal routines can be one way to modulate emotional over-reactivity in the aftermath of a terrorist attack. In the case of the September 11th attack, for example, an attempt to re-establish previous routines within the Falls Church City's school system occurred almost immediately (September 13, 2001). In the case of the snipers, however, normal routines could not be re-established until those responsible were apprehended.

It is also important to understand and utilize the power of symbols as a means of re-establishing community cohesion. For example, following the September 11th terrorist attack, the increased use of the American flag on cars, bridges, trucks, homes, and offices provided individuals with a sense of belonging to "one nation" dedicated to its survival. To fully utilize the power of symbols, it is recommended that organizations, individuals, and governments initiate rituals to honor survivors, rescuers, and the dead through donations and ceremonies (adapted from Everly & Mitchell, 2001).

Guidelines for Children and Families

During the day of September 11, 2001 and the days following, most children were exposed to related images of terror on television and the Internet. Since many of the Washington, DC area schools were closed on Veterans' Day that year, students may have once again been exposed to repeated broadcasts of these images over the course of the day and again on the first anniversary of the attack. Additionally, in the weeks of the sniper crisis, media coverage grew as the snipers expanded their area of terror from Maryland to Richmond (VA). People of all ages in these areas talked about the lack of safety. Mothers pulled into gas stations and "hit the dirt" behind open doors to pump gas. Men placed themselves between gas pumps and car doors to do likewise. The entire

I-95 corridor of traffic became a potential murder scene. An overwhelming sense of relief spread across that area when identification of potential suspects was made. Indeed, within hours parents walked their children to school busses rather than driving them warily to the front doors of schools, and children began to anticipate having recess outside and being able to attend the homecoming football game. The following pages identify major areas for consideration and intervention as school systems attempt to help children deal with community and/or national traumatic events.

Safety. In attempting to ensure that children feel as safe as possible following a community or national trauma, adults need to keep calm and maintain a relaxed, routine environment in both the schools and homes, if at all possible. If the adults cannot stay calm because of personal involvement or loss, then it is important to explain to children why they are upset. This author has found in her professional experience as a school social worker that modeling calmness and control in such situations can serve as emotional cues for children. In addition, adults need to reassure children that every attempt is being made to ensure that they are safe at home, at school, and in the community. Adults also need to demonstrate that they themselves are safe and in control of their own responses to the best of their ability. Furthermore, familiar adults need to remind children of the authorities who are in charge (i.e., law enforcement, fire and rescue, the President, military, teachers) and that these people are trustworthy.

Monitoring behaviors and making referrals. Adults need to examine the children with whom they are in contact for the behavioral and emotional signs of a traumatic stress response, such as sleeplessness, the presence of nightmares, generalized anxiety, and misbehavior. It is important for parents, in particular, to be familiar with emotional states and responses that are age-appropriate in order to give their children reassurance and care, to ask questions or make observations that allow for discussion while remaining tolerant of their children's responses, and to let their children know that feeling upset after such events is normal and acceptable (National Association of School Principals, 2001). According to the APA (2001), helping children talk about their feelings will often also help them to indicate their needs (see also Nader, Pynoos, Fairbanks, & Frederick, 1990; Stevenson, 1992). If children continue to have emotional and/or behavioral problems two months after a traumatic experience, their caregivers can be encouraged to seek out professional help for them.

In addition, it is important to remember that children who are socially close to those who have experienced a disaster (i.e., those whose family members or friends were directly involved or impacted by it) are also quite vulnerable. Children who were only acquainted with a known victim of disaster appear to be somewhat less vulnerable to being traumatized (Nader & Pynoos, 1993; Nisivoccia & Lynn, 1999; Pynoos & Nader, 1989). Similarly, it is also possible for children who identify with the victims of a disaster who are similar in age or citizenship to be traumatized. Responsible adults, therefore, need to make sure that children who appear to be traumatized following a disaster receive the appropriate interventions regardless of the level of their direct involvement. To this end, it is recommended that mental health professionals offer to talk to Parent Teacher Organizations or other organizations about trauma and its healing path. Similarly, they can offer to develop and/or lead trauma-specific counseling groups with the students (Nader & Pynoos, 1993; Nisivoccia & Lynn, 1999; Pynoos & Nader, 1989). Finally, such professionals may also want to offer some sliding scale services to those who cannot afford them or have no insurance during times of crisis.

Monitoring media exposure. It is recommended that parents and other adults monitor the amount and types of media access the children in their care engage in, particularly if they have exhibited trauma-related symptoms. It is important that adults remember to view potentially disturbing images and reports (e.g., broadcasts of the towers collapsing) when children are not around or not awake. This may be difficult, particularly given the continuous coverage that some disastrous events receive. In such cases, it is easy for adults to become victims of what an Australian colleague, Dr. Lenore Meldrum, has termed "CNN-Syndrome" (personal communication, September 13, 2001). In such cases, it is easy for adults to forget how viewing "adult material" can damage an already traumatized or vulnerable child.

Finding meaning. Following a disaster, children are trying to understand what has happened. In an effort to accomplish this goal, they will often make statements or ask questions repetitively. It is important for adults to listen to these communications with respect and respond to them until the child is satisfied. Providing children with the truth about the extent and seriousness of what has occurred, sticking to the facts without dwelling on gruesome details, and using developmentally appropriate language, can help in this process.

During times of crisis, adults and/or parents need to encourage children to be kind to people of all ethnic groups. Similarly, to avoid encouraging discrimination and racism it should be emphasized that violence, hate, and terrorism are the senseless acts of individuals or small groups, not of entire peoples. Therefore, in a series of family/employee meetings held at the World Bank, this author discussed the need for tolerance and helped other bank members provide reassurance to their Islamic colleagues. During such times, it is recommended that parents and other adults discuss the presence of good and evil in the world, particularly with older children and adolescents, in order to help them find meaning in their experience. One way that a child/adolescent can find meaning in a disaster is to take some form of action. Often these actions involve helping others. Therefore, it is recommended that parents/adults encourage children to volunteer in appropriate activities that help the victims of violence. Some volunteer activities that may be appropriate for children to engage in include making drawings for Sesame Street, collecting money, food, and clothing for other victims, writing letters to military personnel, and working as candy stripers. Participating in such actions may help children and adults to gain a sense of purpose and meaning, give them a way to cope through action, and enhance their feelings of self-worth because they are doing something to help others.

Parental/Adult Responses

Parents and other adults respond to terrorism within the community based on their own psychological, physical, emotional, and spiritual characteristics, as well as their previous experiences and personal traits. Parents should, therefore, look at how the events have affected their own personal lives and activities and consider the impact that subsequent travel and separations from their families will have on their children.

When assessing children's needs for intervention, adults need to keep in mind how vulnerable they are to experiencing adverse reactions. Those children who have experienced direct exposure to the events of September 11th, the sniper attacks, or any other large crisis situation, for example, are the most vulnerable to longer and more severe reactions. Those who were witnesses or who had a near miss experience are next in vulnerability. Those within hearing, feeling, or smelling range of the event, but who did not personally witness what happened, fall next on the vulnerability continuum. Children outside the disaster area are typically least vulnerable (Pynoos & Nader, 1989). The role of the media in recent events, however, may have increased the vulnerability of non-witnessing children to being traumatized, as they frequently witnessed the events repeatedly during the media's subsequent news coverage. Therefore, adults responsible for the well-being of children will need to consider this factor when monitoring a child's need for interventions.

GUIDELINES FOR SCHOOLS

In the midst of any crisis, every public and private school aims to represent a safe, responsive environment that can reassure children of their own personal safety. As part of that endeavor, school systems have many tasks and obligations. To meet this goal, most school systems have created crisis response protocols and teams to deal with the potential problems, both large and small, that can occur within or impact their environment following a tragedy. Although the response of such teams can represent an essential factor in a child's adjustment, it is essential that they do not interfere with tactical assessment and rescue efforts of law enforcement and/or EMS professionals (Everly & Mitchell, 2001). Before any plan can be implemented, therefore, certain policies and procedures must be in place to guide working relationships and roles of the various response team personnel. If a school system has not yet created protocols or established teams, this article may serve as a guideline.

Roles

Those individuals in charge of a school's crisis team (generally the administration) must ensure that personnel can work well together in order to plan and carry out appropriate interventions. Faculty members need to be flexible in allowing crisis team members to come into classrooms as time and availability allows. The superintendent needs to take a supportive role, along with the assistant superintendent, and may decide to stand in the halls of the most impacted school, as the comforting "parental" figure. In some systems, all decisions are made from the "top down"; in others, the building administrator has control and only directly checks in with the central office when necessary or when the situation indicates it is appropriate. It is generally the school administrator, though, who writes letters about crisis responses and events that students take home or who sets the tone for crisis team members acceptance in the building.

In view of these considerations, before trying to implement any part of a plan, crisis team coordinators/leaders need make sure that they have the support of administrators in the school and at the central office. It is important to identify any potential trouble spots or hazards that need immediate intervention and define roles clearly before any the team is actually needed. Role confusion or power struggles between the crisis team and school personnel are likely to impede the usefulness of both during a time of crisis.

Any school crisis plan must be adaptable and flexible, designed to meet specific crises as they arise. The roles of those who belong to the crisis team can also be flexible. Faculty may co-lead debriefings, develop appropriate class activities, and express personal grief during these events. Administrators should remain visible, get appropriate information to the school information/media officials, maintain constant contact with the superintendent and the crisis team, be available to the parents and spouses of the deceased, set up schedules of debriefings and interventions, and chair a community meeting if needed. Crisis coordinators may also need to be on-site, spend time in the community with parents and officials, and act as liaisons between the central office and administrative staff.

Safety and Routine

Schools should train teachers and staff in various aspects of trauma, crisis response, abuse, debriefing, and post-traumatic stress so that all school personnel can help students and themselves cope with and adjust to the aftermath of a crisis. In addition, such training would provide school personnel with the skills needed to help those most impacted by the crisis to re-enter and succeed in the school environment. Ideally, this training should occur before the crisis.

While the primary goal of a school system is education and providing knowledge, it is unethical to expect children to perform at their academic potentials shortly after a traumatic event. In times of crisis, therefore, creating a sense of safety within the school, while maintaining structure and routine as much as is possible, can be more important. Therefore, it is best to limit major tests and projects that might be due shortly after a major traumatic event has occurred. In many instances, those students who have been most directly impacted will need additional support and leniency in academic requirements. Helping them return to a sense of normalcy and routine takes precedence over term papers or examination scores. On the other hand, it is important to know when students need to return to class or academic activities rather than mill around halls or use a crisis as a reason to get attention or just stay out of class. One advantage to using a team "from within" is that members of the team frequently have more than crisis-based information about the students and are more able to recognize when requests for help and intervention are manipulation rather than a true crisis response.

PROVISION OF INFORMATION AND CREATION OF MEANING

Early Responses

Schools frequently are a major source of information for parents and communities during times of crisis, particularly if the crisis has directly impacted or occurred within the school's boundaries. School personnel, particularly office staff, may become inundated with phone calls as soon as word of a crisis gets out. Thinking about what to say ahead of time can help lessen the stress on staff. Thus, it is important to answer all crisis-related phone calls using a prepared response. A sample message is presented in Table 1. Extra staff may be needed to help answer phones; in addition, schools should have a designated individual who will respond to the media.

Information Guidelines

Crisis response team leaders in the schools need to provide information to teachers (and parents) as to what to say to children and how to answer their questions, and then give examples of ways to provide that information as they attempt to resolve children's distress. Within the school system itself, information should be given using school staff members in person rather than using public address systems or other media.

TABLE 1. Sample Outgoing Phone Message During a Crisis

You have reached [*school name*] on [*date*].

[*State the general nature of the problem: death of a student/staff member, bomb threat, bus accident, etc.*] All staff members are currently working on this situation and we cannot take your phone call right now. Phone lines must be kept open.

[*If there is a safety emergency, then add the following sentence:*] All necessary measures are being implemented to ensure student safety, which is our top priority. Please do not come to the school building. Students will be sent home with written information for parents. Thank you for your patience and cooperation.

[*You might also add:*] Each school building has a crisis management plan that will help staff deal with the situation and will maintain student safety. Please turn to Media General Cable Channel [*if one is available*] for important information [*or direct the caller to a school Web site*].

Early elementary school children need brief, simple information balanced with reassurances of safety and structure. The extent of family disruption is often an indicator of the young child's degree of upset. The information provided should help them make sense of what happened. Older elementary and early middle school aged children tend to ask more questions about safety and interventions. They are more aware of potential dangers around them and are more active in their search for order. They may have some difficulty understanding how and why humans do such horrible things to one another and have active imaginations that stir up fears and anxiety reactions. They tend to have more somatic complaints and regressive behaviors or school reluctance. Upper middle and high school aged students have strong opinions that can vary greatly. They may have concrete suggestions for interventions and can make commitments to do things to help victims and communities. They may need to appear competent during this time and may lose faith in those around them, particularly if those adults appear weak. They may develop depression or may socially withdraw in response to crisis. In most instances, their symptoms do not persist over extended time periods.

School-based Activities and Interventions

As previously stated, school crisis team leaders need to be able to provide appropriate information to teachers, students, and parents after a critical incident occurs. This information might include what to say to children, how to answer questions children might pose, and ways to help children resolve immediate and more long-term distress. In some situations, the only response made might be a letter sent home with the child. If the trauma occurred during school hours or to a school member (staff or student), someone from the trauma team needs to be in the classroom(s) when announcements are made. The announcement provides students and staff with factual information that is accurate and age appropriate. As new facts become known, updating information and including as much detail as is determined to be appropriate is also important to quell potential rumors.

Types of Interventions

Before crisis intervention activities are implemented, crisis team members (working with the administrators in charge) must decide what type of intervention to use. Possible choices include: (a) defusings; (b) debriefings; (c) large group meetings; and (d) parent information meetings. A defusing occurs very shortly after the traumatic incident in a one-on-one conversation that is designed to discuss the incident and obtain some objective support, generally from a peer (Mitchell & Everly, 1993). When teachers, administrators, pupil personnel staff members, and other school staff process a traumatic event prior to interacting with students, they frequently defuse the situation for one another. The key aspects of defusing are promptness, proximity to the incident, positive atmosphere, brevity, simplicity, and expectancy of recovery (Snelgrove, 1998).

An educational debriefing frequently takes place prior to intervening with students and/or families. Thus, it is important for crisis team members, central office staff, and administrators to meet with staff as soon as is possible after the trauma; if the event occurred the night before or after school ended, then meet the first thing in the morning. The facts are set straight during this debriefing and members plan what to tell students, parents, and others. Schools that have a phone tree should begin this intervention even before this meeting.

When the word "debriefing" is used, it generally refers to a psychological and educational group process designed to mitigate the impact of a critical incident (Mitchell & Everly, 1993). A debriefing is not a therapy session, nor is it an investigation of what happened or a critique of process or procedure. It is a structured group process designed to help individuals examine and review their personal experiences resulting from or dealing with the critical incident.

There are numerous models of debriefing. However, all models have a series of stages that begin with a discussion of the more factual and rationally based information (i.e., what happened) before proceeding into a discussion of the more emotional issues (e.g., how one was impacted by what happened, what was considered to be the worst part of the event) and the symptoms that the event might engender. The debriefing will then return to a more rationally based stage that includes teaching and closure activities. Guidelines for who should require debriefing include the following: (a) debrief those with the greatest need first; (b) try to keep debriefing groups homogeneous (children of the same age or in the same class); and (c) observe symptoms during the debriefing without pushing anyone to participate (Mitchell & Everly, 1993).

If the decision is to use debriefings, a discussion of the students' and staff's factual knowledge, reactions at the time of the event through present time, and feelings then and now surrounding the crisis event should ensue. The debriefing process usually lasts between 15-60 minutes, depending on the age and stage of the students. Preschool-kindergarten debriefings last between 15-30 minutes; elementary debriefings, between 30 minutes and 1 hour; middle school debriefings, between 45 minutes and 1 1/2 hours; high school debriefings, between 1 and 2 hours, or longer if needed. It is important to allow for smaller group sessions and/or individual sessions if/when needed (Johnson, 1993).

In doing the debriefings, it is important to be aware of community aspects of the events, the nature of the community, key themes of the event and community reactions, organization issues, power struggles within the organization and community, and interpersonal relationships. Another aspect of the debriefing involves a discussion of the meaning of what happened while providing students with information about potential reactions in the future. Education is a major function of the debriefing and information should be delivered in a way that is easy for participants to comprehend. If necessary, particularly with younger children, the debriefing can include art or other activities that help participants to process the information being discussed and express themselves.

It is not just the student body that may need to be debriefed. It may also be important to debrief the faculty, members of the crisis team and parents, particularly when they show signs of compassion fatigue and/or being overwhelmed. These debriefing sessions may need to be held after school and into the evening to accommodate the schedules of these adults. Schools should be encouraged to utilize outside help if a trained team is available, as it is not advisable for the team to debrief itself.

Other Interventions

It will be important to identify individuals who are most impacted by the crisis and who need a more individualized approach. Inevitably, some students will need closer attention and supervision than others. In such instances, it may be important to assign staff members to remain in the various locations where students congregate. It can also be important to staff "drop in" centers that are available for students, faculty, and staff members who need counseling.

School staff members should also plan for potential interventions after the immediate response if students have been absent or have been directly injured or impacted by the event. These students may heal at a different rate than those involved in school activities shortly after the event occurred.

It is also important for crisis team leaders and administration to develop trauma specific resources and materials to be used during classroom discussions and activities. Alternative activities introduced in the classroom that involve writing or drawing about what happened can facilitate this processing. According to Poland and McCormick (1999), drawings can help faculty members understand how students "perceive what happened during the crisis and can facilitate conversation about how they are coping" (p. 184). Asking students to explain what their artwork says offers them the opportunity to ventilate and express emotions, ideas, and impacts. For example, following the September 11th terrorist attacks, first grade students at H. Byron Masterson Elementary School (2002) wrote and illustrated a book about how the events of that day impacted them. Their artwork depicted the events of September 12, 2001 and indicated that, on that day, they knew "everything would be all right" (p. 6).

Students of all ages can portray thoughts, emotions, somatic responses, beliefs, and other traumatic impacts through artwork. Themes of that work could range from their role or experience during an event to their perception of the victims to what the event means to them and how to commemorate what happened. If students do not want to draw their response, they might do a collage, create a sculpture, or build an artifact symbolic of what happened.

Another way to incorporate what happened into classroom activities is to introduce literary passages and works that portray disaster, trauma, grief, reactivity, resilience, and triumph. Various organizations have compiled booklists on topics related to trauma; for example, the Association of Traumatic Stress Specialists (ATSS) is one such organization. Students can also be encouraged or assigned to develop poetry, essays, research papers, journal entries, or other literary works as another means to deal with their own traumatic reactions. Further, students may be given writing assignments that relate to a traumatic event. Reiss (2002, p. 151) suggests the following assignments: (a) write the worst thing that ever happened to you; (b) write about your most scary nightmare; (c) write about how you felt when you first heard the news of a traumatic event; (d) write about how you feel now that the event is over; (e) write about your life as it is now; and (f) write about what others have said about what happened.

Additional activities might be designed to teach tolerance and avoid the stereotyping of specific groups, nationalities, or victim groups to mitigate the occurrence of later violence against perceived perpetrators. School staff members might also interact with various community organizations to develop community-based activities as outlets. Schools can also make age-appropriate reading materials available to persons beyond the school walls by providing handouts at parent informational meetings and community activities.

TEACH CHILDREN TO MAKE LISTS

Reiss (2002) notes, "making lists can be therapeutic to those in mourning" (p. 63). Teaching and encouraging children of all ages to make lists (e.g., lists of things to do, lists of things that have been impacted by what happened, lists of things that have not changed, lists of things children like about themselves) can build normalcy and create a sense of focus and grounding. Lists can be future-oriented, thereby re-orienting children to something beyond the past traumatic event and the pain of the present. Lists, therefore, can influence the sense of foreshortened future that many children experience after a traumatic event. They can also encourage the child to search for meaning in what has happened or can help build the child's sense of resilience. For example, a list of "things for which I am thankful" can help develop a more positive post-event attitude. Children can also take the assignment home and share it with parents/caregivers as a way to encourage positive thought in the family.

SCHOOL BASED ACTIVITIES DEALING WITH TRAUMATIC GRIEF

It is possible that those most impacted by a death, particularly one that has been traumatic, may never fully accept the loss of the deceased. However, dealing with that death in a school system may help facilitate closure, as well as an acceptance of the death as being real and final, and may even lead to some sense of reconciliation (Wolfelt, 1987). Thus, grief-based groups led by counselors, psychologists, or school social workers can help students achieve Worden's (1991) tasks of grieving, which include: (a) accepting the reality of the death; (b) experiencing the pain and anguish of grief; (c) adjusting to the world in which the deceased is no longer present in the physical sense; and (d) moving on with life, putting the deceased into his/her new role or position.

Children who have lost significant individuals through death, particularly a traumatic death, may feel isolated and alone in their grief. Support groups can provide such students with guidance and an emotional outlet as a way to combat that isolation in a supportive atmosphere, and can be an important role of school personnel. The objectives of groups include: (a) provision of information about the process and tasks of grief; (b) provision of a forum to express emotions and concerns about the grief process and personal experiences; (c) inclusion of structured activities to assist in working through grief (e.g., activities looking at how the death has changed their lives, anger and guilt based activities, commemorative activities, and mixed media activities); (d) examination of current support systems and ways to use those systems or expand them if they are ineffective; and (e) development of a resource base of materials as well as peers (Perschy, 1997).

Young (1996) suggests numerous intervention methods and strategies that could be adapted to a grief group. These include oral storytelling, sometimes with the leader providing the initial sentence of the story; discussion based on a particularly poignant photo, poem, or video; creative writing of poems, memory books, journal entries; creative art projects; dramatic presentations (making a puppet theater for younger children or writing a play for older students); or craft projects such as creating personalized worry beads.

TRAUMA-BASED GROUPS ORIENTED TO RESILIENCE AND COPING

The trauma-based group goes beyond the grief-focused group and deals with specific symptoms of post-traumatic stress disorder (PTSD), including intrusive thoughts, nightmares, avoidance activities, startle responses, and others (Nisivoccia & Lynn, 1999). Such groups provide a venue to express fear, share humorous (even black humor) stories, gain information from others with more factual knowledge of what happened or will happen, and learn about each other's experiences. Ideally, groups have between six and eight members, although a group of 10 to 12 is feasible. Children may rotate, as leaders and/or helpers, choosing the topic for the following week or an activity to use with the chosen topic. Group leaders may or may not ask the students in attendance to share "the story" of what happened to each of them during or with a trauma. They may also be asked to write out, describe, draw, collage, or otherwise represent the worst aspect of what happened, the best aspect, the losses, or other topics. They may also create trigger books of things that they concurrently smell, see, hear, touch, taste or otherwise experience that remind them of the past event(s) (Nisivoccia & Lynn, 1999).

According to their age and developmental stage, students can do various feelings-related activities ranging from making feeling charts to encouraging discussion of ways to modulate feelings (Gordon, Farberow, & Maida, 1999). Whatever the assignment, children need to experience an increased sense of post-event power through provision of options of ways to complete an assignment (Reiss, 2002). One possible group format is based on Schab's (1996) book *The Coping Skills Workbook*. This eleven-week group would begin with an introductory session and then use each of the nine coping skills in the workbook as a topic. Among the coping skills highlighted in the workbook are dealing with feelings, adjusting attitudes, and discovering choices.

INCORPORATE STRESS MANAGEMENT INTO SCHOOL ACTIVITIES AND PROGRAMS

Teachers and counselors can incorporate specific stress reduction activities into the school day. For example, beginning the elementary school day with deep breathing and stretching for five minutes is one such strategy. Teachers can model these exercises while experiencing their relaxing benefits themselves. According to Mendler (1990), relaxation exercises can also be incorporated into times when students are transitioning between high stress and energy activities (e.g., recess, physical education) and focused classroom activities (e.g., one of the core subjects).

NOTIFICATIONS

School personnel should notify any other schools that are impacted (e.g., schools of siblings if there was a death of a student; former students if there was a death of teacher), as well as "latchkey" parents whose children are without parental presence when first arriving home from school. These children may need their parents to come home early to provide support following a crisis. At the end of the first day, schools may wish to send a newsletter or flyer home with every student that describes what happened, what the school did to intervene post-crisis, what constitutes a normal post-traumatic stress reaction, and answers to the questions that family members are likely to have. The flier also can provide information about what questions to ask and what information to provide, as well as how to help children (and themselves) through the grief process. It is also important to keep school board members, administration (central office), and community officials fully informed of the school's response and notify them immediately of any unsuspected outcomes or information that might be learned (e.g., copycat suicide pacts).

POST EVENT ACTIVITIES AND INTERVENTIONS

In the event of the death of a student or staff member, certain decisions need to be made. One decision is whether or not to gather up personal effects of the deceased from lockers, desks, and classroom. This can be very controversial. In some instances, a "shrine" may spontaneously develop in the classroom. In other cases, students may want to have a "shrine" somewhere else in the building. Schools should have a pre-existing policy in place regarding the existence of such memorials, as well as the parameters and time limits for such shrines if they are allowed. If the victim was a teacher, schools should take time to dispose of that teacher's personal effects in the classroom. Also, staff and students should be allowed to decide on appropriate school-based or school sponsored commemorative rituals and discuss those plans with the family.

It is additionally important to be in touch with family members about such arrangements and whether or not they want a small, private viewing and/or service or a large wake and/or service that include students and staff. If the wake is to have an open coffin, schools should notify parents as soon as possible; this will allow parents time to discuss death and the presentation of dead bodies with their children and/or make informed decisions whether their children will attend. It may also be wise to have crisis team members available at both the wake and the funeral for those who have a need for immediate assistance. If the response to a funeral is going to be very large, the suggestion might be for the funeral to be held on a non-school day (e.g., Saturday). If this is not possible or not desired, then it may be necessary to arrange for substitutes to cover classrooms and busses to take students and faculty to the funeral, pending parental permission.

If staff members anticipate that large numbers of students will attend the funeral, and there will be special circumstances at that commemoration, it is also important to let parents and other staff know ahead of time so that potential crisis reactions can be prevented or dealt with. For example, following the suicide of an eighth grade student who was Greek Orthodox, the traditional funeral practice held by the family involved having everyone in the congregation view the body and touch, kiss, or display affection to it. Many students who attended this service were overwhelmed and needed crisis intervention immediately, as did some of the staff and parents in attendance. In such situations, it may also be important to have persons available to staff and students who remain at school during a funeral because they cannot, will not, or are not permitted to attend the services but have been impacted by the individual's death.

REFERRALS

Schools are generally closed systems that prefer to determine their own crisis responses. However, if the schools have good working relationships with local mental health professionals or trained trauma specialists, then those persons may be included in school crisis plans or as potential referral sources for traumatized students and staff members. School counselors are generally the first level of intervention for the most distressed or symptomatic students. Accordingly, school counselors should develop lists of available community referral sources that specialize in the treatment of trauma; referrals can then be provided to students and parents when there is concern about the level of distress that a student displays.

REVIEW AND EVALUATION

It is also important to evaluate the team's response and its successes and failures following an intervention. This evaluation allows the team to better plan for the next crisis and to revise its protocol, if necessary. When making this evaluation, the following questions should be considered: (a) how much disequilibria still exists in the school; (b) how much organizational confusion still exists; (c) how well did team members do their jobs; (d) how well were emotions defused; (e) did rumors and myths get addressed and corrected; and (f) was healthy, adaptive coping stressed and then implemented?

WHAT MIGHT SCHOOL PERSONNEL FEEL DURING AND AFTER A CRISIS?

School staff members often feel a variety of emotions and have a variety of responses after a school crisis. They may feel helpless, realizing there is little they can do to change the situation, to bring back the deceased, to heal the grief of witnesses or those closely connected to the person(s) who died. They may feel fearful or anxious as well as vulnerable after they have been exposed to a trauma and its impact. For example, seeing the death of a child can shatter the illusion of invulnerability, lower self-efficacy, and weaken the belief in an internal locus of control. In addition, some school staff members become fearful that something similar could occur in their own families or in the families of their loved ones, thus increasing their sense of personal vulnerability.

Some staff members experience rage and anger toward those who may be seen as responsible for the traumatic incident. This rage and anger may lead to intolerance and a lack of trust in others. Others may feel intense sorrow and grief. They could consequently experience intrusive images of the traumatic events, particularly surrounding the death of a child. Mental images of the scene (e.g., the collapse of the Twin Towers) come back intensely and often unbidden. Still other staff members may feel some degree of self-reproach and shame, particularly if they are questioning what they could have done differently to prevent the event from occurring. They may experience a change in values or appreciation of their own families. The helping educator may appreciate life more. Finding escape in humor is less useful when children are involved and does not seem to reduce tension, keep emotional distance, or build cohesion and morale in situations in which there is a death of a child. Thus, this defense mechanism is less available to protect (Dyregrov & Mitchell, 1992).

Because emotions and reactions may run rampant during and after a traumatic event, it is essential that school systems establish programs and opportunities for staff self-care. Initial debriefings of crisis team members are essential, preferably run by someone outside the system who has distance from the actual event. After one such event involving the deaths of two students in unrelated incidents, the Superintendent of Schools in Falls Church (VA), Mary Ellen Shaw, took the entire crisis team and administrative staff out to lunch after that debriefing. Bringing in wellness consultants, setting up wellness related activities on a professional day, and encouraging social activities and other such events may be particularly helpful to decrease these emotions and return a sense of homeostasis.

FINAL THOUGHTS

Given the events in our nation and our schools over the past several years, one thing is now clearer to us than ever before: the next school crisis that occurs could be in your area. School crises of a variety of types can happen anywhere at any time, and no two crises are ever alike. The mental health of our nation's children should be of utmost concern. However, too many children still have no health insurance, and mental health clinics still have long waiting lists. In addition, finding qualified traumatologists is not an easy matter, particularly those willing to operate on a sliding scale fee system or do pro bono work. It is also clear that all members of a school community will be impacted by a tragedy regardless of the role that they play within the school system. Therefore, it is essential for both students and helping personnel to take time for themselves and to talk about their feelings. It may also be critical to remember that out of darkness comes light, and out of horror comes hope and resilience. Survival from a traumatic event is not always a straight-line path; it can be difficult, but with help and support it can be done.

REFERENCES

American Psychological Association Disaster Response Network. (2001, September). *Guidelines for helping children deal with terrorism.* Washington, DC: APA.

Bloom, S. (2001, September 16). *Message to the membership of the International Society of Traumatic Stress Studies.* Retrieved from, www.ISTSS.com.

Dyregrov, A., & Mitchell, J. T. (1992). Working with traumatized children: Psychological effects and coping strategies. *Journal of Traumatic Stress, 5*(1), 5-17.

Everly, G. S., & Mitchell, J. T. (2001, Summer). America under attack: The "10 Commandments" of responding to mass terrorist attacks. *International Journal of Emergency Mental Health, 3*(3), 133-135.

Gordon, N. S., Farberow, N. L., & Maida, C. A. (1999). *Children & disasters.* Philadelphia, PA: Brunner-Mazel.

H. Byron Masterson Elementary School First Grade Class. (2002). *September 12th we knew everything would be all right.* New York: Scholastic, Inc.

Johnson, K. (1993). *Trauma in the lives of children: Crisis and stress management techniques for teachers, counselors, and student service professionals.* Alameda, CA: Hunter House Books.

Mendler, A. N. (1990). *Smiling at yourself: Educating young children about stress and self-esteem.* Santa Cruz, CA: Network Publications.

Mitchell, J. T., & Everly, G. S. (1993). *Critical incident stress debriefing: An operations manual for the prevention of trauma among emergency service and disaster workers.* Baltimore, MD: Chevron Press.

Myers, D. (2001, August). *Terrorism as a special type of crisis.* Paper presented at the annual meeting of the American Psychological Association, San Francisco, CA.

Nader, K., & Pynoos, R. (1993). School disaster: Planning and initial interventions. *Journal of Social Behavior and Personality, 8*(5), 299-320.

Nader, K., Pynoos, R. S., Fairbanks, L., & Frederick, C. (1990). Children's PTSD reactions one year after a sniper attack at their school. *American Journal of Psychiatry, 147*, 1526-1530.

National Association of School Principals. (2001, September). *Guidelines for parents: Helping your children deal with terrorism.* Bethesda, MD: Author.

Nisivoccia, D., & Lynn, M. (1999). Helping forgotten victims: Using activities groups with children who witness violence. In N. B. Webb (Ed.), *Play therapy with children in crisis: Individual, group, and family treatment* (2nd ed., pp. 74-103). New York: The Guilford Press.

Perschy, M. K. (1997). *Helping teens work through grief.* Washington, DC: Accelerated Development.

Poland, S., & McCormick, J. S. (1999). *Coping with crisis, lessons learned: A resource for schools, parents, and communities.* Longmont, CO: Sopris West.

Pynoos, R. S., & Nader, K. O. (1989). Children's memory and proximity to violence. *Journal of the American Academy of Child and Adolescent Psychiatry, 28,* 236-241.

Reiss, F. (2002). *Terrorism and kids: Comforting your child.* Newton, MA: Peanut Butter and Jelly Press.

Schab, L. M. (1996). *The coping skills workbook: Teaches kids nine essential skills to help deal with real-life crises.* King of Prussia, PA: The Center for Applied Psychology, Inc.

Shaw, M. E. (2001, September 20). Superintendent reports on schools crisis response. *Falls Church News Press, XI* (28), 2, 19.

Snelgrove, T. (1998, March). *Managing acute traumatic stress: Trauma interventor's resource manual, 11th ed.* West Vancouver, BC: Easton-Snelgrove, Ind.

Stevenson, R. G. (1992). Sudden death in schools. In N. B. Webb (Ed.), *Helping bereaved children: A handbook for practitioners* (pp. 194-213). New York: The Guilford Press.

Wolfelt, A. (1987, Winter). Resolution versus reconciliation: The importance of semantics. *Thanatos, 12,* 10-13.

Worden, J. W. (1991). *Grief counseling and grief therapy* (2nd ed.). New York: Springer Publishing Company.

Young, M. A. (1996, August). *Working with grieving children after violent death: A guidebook for crime victim assistance professionals.* Washington, DC: United States Department of Justice Office for Victims of Crime.

The Forensic Examination
of Posttraumatic Stress Disorder

Chrys J. Harris

SUMMARY. The diagnosis of posttraumatic stress disorder (PTSD) has achieved a major level of significance in our judicial system. The forensic examination of PTSD is identified as a specialized assessment that is non-biased and non-prejudicial. This article attempts to provide a standard methodology to offer an objective and neutral forensic assessment and diagnosis of PTSD that will stand up to legal scrutiny by identifying problems in diagnosing PTSD and establishing a six-step methodology for the differential diagnosis of the disorder. Procedures for providing a forensic examination of PTSD and details of the author's methods of providing a forensic examination are presented. *[Article copies available for a fee from The Haworth Document Delivery Service: 1-800-HAWORTH. E-mail address: <docdelivery@haworthpress.com> Website: <http://www.HaworthPress.com> © 2006 by The Haworth Press, Inc. All rights reserved.]*

KEYWORDS. Posttraumatic Stress Disorder, PTSD, forensic examination, forensics

---

Address correspondence to Chrys J. Harris, Family Therapy & Trauma Center, 311 Bennett Center Drive, Greer, SC 29650 (E-mail: chrysharris@traumacenter.biz).

The author would like to acknowledge Charles R. Figley, PhD (Florida State University), for his chiasmal fascination with traumatic stress. Without his interest, the author would have none.

[Haworth co-indexing entry note]: "The Forensic Examination of Posttraumatic Stress Disorder." Harris, Chrys J. Co-published simultaneously in *Journal of Aggression, Maltreatment & Trauma* (The Haworth Maltreatment & Trauma Press, an imprint of The Haworth Press, Inc.) Vol. 12, No. 1/2, 2006, pp. 83-102; and: *Trauma Treatment Techniques: Innovative Trends* (ed: Jacqueline Garrick, and Mary Beth Williams) The Haworth Maltreatment & Trauma Press, an imprint of The Haworth Press, Inc., 2006, pp. 83-102. Single or multiple copies of this article are available for a fee from The Haworth Document Delivery Service [1-800-HAWORTH, 9:00 a.m. - 5:00 p.m. (EST). E-mail address: docdelivery@haworthpress.com].

doi:10.1300/J146v12n01_05

83

PTSD has become a growth industry. No diagnosis in American psychiatry has had such a profound influence on civil and criminal law.

Simon, 1995a, p. xv

The diagnosis of posttraumatic stress disorder (PTSD) has achieved a major level of significance in our judicial system. PTSD is a mental health disorder that often develops following exposure to a traumatic event that is experienced as potentially life threatening for one's self or one's significant other(s). Three characteristic symptom clusters of this disorder include symptoms associated with re-experiencing of the event, symptoms associated with increased arousal, and symptoms associated with avoidance or numbing (van der Kolk & McFarlane, 1996).

The prevalence of PTSD diagnoses that are deliberated in courtrooms all over the country has become so considerable it has prompted Frances, First, and Pincus (1995) to suggest that this diagnosis may be overused in litigation. Regardless of whether the diagnosis is overused, used correctly, or misused, it has become a major consideration in civil law and, to a lesser extent, in criminal law. The principal reason that PTSD has become such a prominent part of the judicial system involves the fact that it can be directly related to a traumatic incident in a relationship that implies causation and culpability for the emotional symptoms that follow.

The domain in which the mental health field and the legal system overlap involves the use of expert witnesses, and requires exactness and a freedom from errors in the diagnosis of any physical or mental disorder, including PTSD. Those who are finders of fact (i.e., usually juries and judges) demand accuracy to ensure their conclusions and verdicts are based on certainty rather than conjecture. Therefore, the forensic identification and diagnosis of PTSD can be seen as an endeavor to provide the finders of fact with such certainty.

Matson (1999) defined an expert witness as "a person who, by reasons of education or special training, possesses knowledge of some particular subject area in greater depth than the public at large" (p. 17). To be included as evidence, Matson suggests the expert's testimony must: (a) establish the facts; (b) interpret the facts, usually in the form of an opinion; (c) comment on the opposing expert's testimony or opinion; and (d) define customary professional standards in the expert's area of qualification. These four expectations of an expert's testimony differentiate it from the testimony offered by the witnesses and principle parties involved in a legal case. So how is a forensic expert delineated from other experts?

The word *forensic* derives from the Roman concept of a forum, literally meaning a public discussion (Babitsky; Mangraviti & Todd, 2000). A forensic expert is commonly a specialist in a specific scientific field. As such, the forensic expert brings science and the law together by offering a legally acceptable scientific opinion. In the American culture of the immediate past, portrayals of the forensic field have primarily had to do with medical examiners and their work with the deceased. In fact, many Americans defined a forensic scientist as being similar to the character Jack Klugman played on the television series *Quincy, M.E.* (Larson, 1976). However, in the past few years, television has introduced a new forensic specialist to the American public, that of the crime scene investigator on series such as *CSI* (Zuiker et al., 2000). Medical examiners (like Quincy) and crime scene investigators (like the characters on *CSI*) are, indeed, forensic scientists. However, forensic scientists can be found in almost any field. In fact, Edwards (1998) suggested that the American court system presently uses forensic experts from over 3,000 disciplines (e.g., forensic accountants, forensic engineers, and forensic social workers). They bring their scientific principles, practices, and ethical standards to bear on civil and criminal matters as forensic expert witnesses.

Although a clinical therapist can be an expert witness, there are some distinct differences between the clinical examination that most therapists perform and a typical forensic examination. Greenfield (1999) has suggested four parameters that illustrate the contrast (see Table 1). In the first parameter, the purpose of the forensic examination is to investigate and offer an opinion regarding the inquiry. Although this opinion usually centers on a diagnostic impression, there can be other motives for a PTSD forensic examination (e.g., to determine if the examinee is malingering, or to assess for the continuing need for treatment [duration and cost]). In fact, any concern the legal system may have regarding an individual ostensibly diagnosed with PTSD could be a potential focus for forensic examination.

The second parameter proposed by Greenfield suggests that advocacy in a forensic analysis is neutral and oriented solely towards acquiring the necessary opinion. In fact, developing a neutral, unbiased, unprejudiced, objective opinion that is fair and impartial in nature is probably the *sine qua non* for a forensic inquiry. Alternatively, in a clinical setting, most therapists and counselors are advocates for their clients.

TABLE 1. Distinctions Between a Clinical and a Forensic Examination

PARAMETER	CLINICAL EXAMINATION	FORENSIC EXAMINATION
Purpose	Assessment and treatment	Inquiry and opinion
Advocacy	For the Examinee (biased)	For the Opinion (neutral)
Scope	Multiple sessions/hours	Limited to a few sessions/hours
Examinee's perception of the examiner	Advocate	1. Examination for the *examinee*–advocate 2. Examination for the *other side*–adversary
Confidentiality	Provisions of State/Federal law	Limited provisions of law

Greenfield's third parameter suggests that the Independent Medical Examination (IME) for Emotional Trauma of the examinee is not fundamentally a long-term event, and should therefore be limited in a forensic examination. Although the amount of time needed to reach the required opinion may actually take much longer than the time allowed for an IME for Emotional Trauma (due to the examination of collateral observers, other knowing parties, relevant documents, and other significantly related materials), the actual time spent with an examinee is limited to the time required to perform the necessary IME for Emotional Trauma in a forensic examination. Therapy or counseling, however, involves time spent with the patient that can go on indefinitely.

Finally, the fourth parameter described by Greenfield identifies the examiner as an advocate only if the forensic examination is being performed at the request of the examinee's attorney. On the other hand, if the forensic examination is being performed at the request of the opposing side or the court, the examiner will usually be viewed as an adversary by the examinee. Obviously, how the forensic examiner is perceived by the examinee is paramount for client anxiety, support, truthfulness, and general cooperation.

The fifth parameter presented in Table 1 concerns issues of confidentiality and was included by the present author. Although there is a necessity for informed consent prior to being examined either forensically or clinically, the extent that the client's responses will be confidential differs significantly. In a forensic examination, the finding (i.e., opinion) of the examiner is going to be read potentially by lawyers, a judge, perhaps a jury of peers, and any others who may have standing in the case. In addition, it will also more than likely be discussed openly in a courtroom filled with the public in attendance. As a result, the disclosure statement (i.e., informed consent) for a forensic examination needs to be different from that obtained in traditional therapy. It needs to fully explain to the examinee that his/her statements are not considered confidential and will be released to both sides of the litigation. Although confidentiality and privilege are limited, forensic examiners should observe informed consent rules; in addition, the examinees need to receive some type of disclosure statement identifying the risks of the examination and describing the rights and immunities that they do have (e.g., duties to warn and applicable laws regarding subpoenas and records).

DIAGNOSING PTSD IN A FORENSIC EXAMINATION

Problems. Goldberg (1995) has suggested that hundreds of millions of dollars have been awarded to litigants of civil cases who have claimed psychological injuries. In many of these cases, PTSD was found to be a major factor in determining the outcome of the case. Despite the frequent introduction of PTSD in matters of law, guidelines for the forensic examination of PTSD are varied (Simon, 1995b) and have yet to be standardized. As a result of this variance and lack of standardization, Goldberg (1995) has stated that some PTSD claimants may have been under-compensated for their suffering, while others have been over-compensated. Similarly, it is also possible that some claimants with legitimate diagnoses of PTSD have not received compensation, while others have been compensated for malingering.

To explain the lack of standardization in forensic examinations of PTSD, it is necessary to investigate the inadequate fit between legal concerns and mental health concerns. According to the American Psychiatric Association's (APA; 2000) *Diagnostic and Statistical Manual of Mental Disorders, Fourth Edition, Text Revision* (DSM-IV-TR), obtaining a clinical diagnosis is usually *not* a satisfactory method of establishing a mental health disorder for legal purposes. Indeed, Frances et al. (1995) claimed that the aims and provisions of the *DSM-IV* (APA, 1994) are much different from those of the judicial system. Furthermore, these authors point out that making a diagnosis in a clinical setting is "intended for collegial use in an atmosphere that is very different from the adversarial nature of a typical forensic proceeding" (p. 65). It follows that additional facts supporting the diagnosis are usually required by courts to demonstrate a legal standard. Thus, according to the DSM-IV-TR, the poor fit between the mental health field and the legal system permits clinical information presented in a court case to be utilized unerringly, misused, or misunderstood.

Successful forensic evaluations. Success in the forensic examination of PTSD relies on four components: (a) the expertise of the examiner in both the scientific principles and scientific standards associated with the clinical knowledge of PTSD; (b) the examiner's ability to meet the stipulations and qualifying factors of the legal system, including the guidelines for and specifications of a forensic examination; (c) the examiner's deftness in bringing these components together in an unimpeachable manner; and (d) the examiner's proficiency in testifying convincingly in the courtroom. In other words, the successful PTSD forensic examiner is one who is able to coalesce a proficiency in assessing and treating PTSD with a knowledge of the relevant requirements of the legal system. Additionally, the successful PTSD forensic examiner is one who is not considered a "hired gun" (a term the legal system uses to define any forensic examiner who does only forensics and does not practice within his/her scientific specialty). Successful PTSD forensic examiners maintain a mental health practice concurrent with the forensic practice.

DIFFERENTIAL DIAGNOSIS FOR PTSD

Cooperstein (1999) submitted, "one of the most vexing diagnostic issues to be encountered in psychology is the clinical and forensic identification of . . . PTSD" (p. 18). He aptly conveys a major concern that presently exists in both the field of psychology and in the other professions of mental health. Since PTSD was first introduced in the DSM-III (APA, 1980), clinicians have been struggling to assess and diagnose this disorder accurately. Modlin (1990) wrote, "PTSD in pure form is one of the most specific diagnostic categories in current psychiatric nomenclature, and differential diagnosis poses few problems" (p. 63). Early (1990), however, has suggested that PTSD "is a difficult diagnosis to make with certainty" (p. 137). Regardless of this apparent contradiction, the assessment and diagnosis of PTSD is generally considered to be difficult for a number of reasons.

First and foremost, PTSD is not the only mental health disorder that may result from the exposure to a traumatic stressor. There is evidence, for example, that exposure to a traumatic event can also result in generalized anxiety disorder, panic disorder (with or without agoraphobia), and depression (Modlin, 1990; Resnick, 1997). Furthermore, van der Kolk stated that there is an "intimate association among trauma, dissociation, and somatization" (as cited in van der Kolk & McFarlane, 1996, p. 18), which suggests that the diagnostic categories of dissociative disorders and somatization disorders should not be overlooked when diagnosing someone following exposure to a traumatic event. The DSM-IV-TR (2000) also cautions against making a diagnosis of PTSD without first looking for preexisting disorders that may have been exacerbated by the traumatic experience, opening up the entire gamut of mental health disorders as possible consequences of a traumatic experience. The idea that many, if not all, mental health disorders may result from traumatic events has been supported by McKenzie (2001), who claimed that the source for all serious mental health disorders is actually PTSD/Delayed Onset. The difficulty in measuring or assessing PTSD represents another reason why this diagnosis remains difficult. In fact, there is a multitude of emotional trauma assessment techniques and devices currently on the market (c.f., Carlson, 1997; Stamm, 1996). The quandary for these assessment techniques involves gathering information concerning the examinee's experiences, ostensibly from the client, regarding the traumatic event without having the client provide erroneous information (e.g., faking the disorder or enhancing symptomology). There is only one measure on the market that actually provides a clinical diagnosis for PTSD: the Detailed Assessment of Posttraumatic Stress (DAPS; Briere, 2001). Briere reported that internal consistency (Cronbach's $\pm$) for the clinical scales ranged from .82 to .88, and that scores on the DAPS correlated highly ($r = .87$) with scores obtained on the Clinician-Administered PTSD Scale (CAPS).

The forensic examiner may face a third difficulty related to making the PTSD diagnosis acceptable in a courtroom. The Daubert challenge (*Daubert v. Merrell Dow Pharmaceuticals, Inc.*, 1993) can be used to limit or completely block a forensic examiner's testimony. When a motion *in limine* is filed, suggesting the forensic examiner is not using scientifically valid methods, the judge may convene a hearing to determine whether the underlying reasoning of the forensic examiner's opinion regarding PTSD is scientifically valid and can be properly applied to the facts before the court. This hearing is conducted away from the jury. During this procedure, the judge will consider the following five questions about PTSD: (a) have the theories or techniques regarding PTSD been tested; (b) has PTSD been subjected to peer review and publication; (c) is there a known or potential error rate in the diagnosis of

PTSD; (d) are there standards that control the operation of PTSD; and (e) is there widespread acceptance of PTSD within the relevant scientific community? To survive a Daubert challenge, therefore, the forensic examiner must use appropriate methodologies, standards, and practices, which are known to guarantee that the forensic opinion is derived from and constitutes a form of specialized knowledge by those who commonly work with PTSD.[1] As such, a PTSD diagnosis must meet rigorous legal standards to be used during the course of a legal proceeding.

SIX-STEP MODEL FOR DIFFERENTIALLY DIAGNOSING PTSD

To address the assessment problems and co-morbid diagnoses identified in the literature, First, Frances, and Pincus (1995) have recommended a six-step process for making any differential diagnosis. Through the adaptation of these six steps, a standardized, staged model for diagnosing PTSD can be established, which can be used to reach a credible forensic differential diagnosis. Although each step is presented and defined herein, a description of the actual methods used to accomplish each of the proposed steps is beyond the scope of this article.

Step 1. The first step proposed by First et al. (1995) involves ruling out malingering and/or factitious disorders. This initial step in the differential diagnosis process is of paramount importance to ensure that a credible forensic diagnosis is obtained. The DSM-IV (APA, 1994) defines malingering as:

> the intentional production of false or grossly exaggerated physical or psychological symptoms, motivated by external incentives such as avoiding military duty, avoiding work, obtaining financial compensation, evading criminal prosecution, or obtaining drugs. (p. 683)

It is this author's suggestion that malingering should be strongly suspected if there is an attorney referral for a forensic examination, whether medical or emotional. Indeed, attorneys (from one side or the other) usually engage the forensic examiner, making attorney referrals the norm. Additionally, with the field of forensics playing a more extensive role in judicial proceedings, malingering should also be strongly suspected if the client is self-referred for a forensic examination. This is because a plaintiff may attempt to use the forensic examination to potentially prove non-existent emotional distress in order to obtain the large sums that juries often award for emotional damage. Resnick (1997) has suggested that PTSD, unlike any other diagnosis in the DSM-IV (APA, 1994), demonstrates a causal link between a traumatic incident and what may be, in essence, a compensable mental health problem. For example, Resnick claimed that unlike PTSD, Acute Stress Disorder (ASD), which also results from exposure to a traumatic event and involves PTSD-like symptomology, is unlikely to be malingered due to its limited time frame (i.e., two days to four weeks). As such, forensic examiners should be cautioned to expect a predisposition for examinees to malinger when being evaluated for PTSD, specifically when such a diagnosis would add to a financial judgment in litigation.

Factitious Disorder, on the other hand, is somewhat less problematic for the forensic examiner because, according to the DSM-IV-TR (APA, 2000), the examinee that might have this mental health problem is looking to take on the role of an ailing person. This disorder is distinguished from malingering in that the motivation for feigning distress is an emotional, albeit pathological, need to take on a sick role rather than to achieve an external incentive. Since the incentive is internal, those who have a factitious disorder do not usually go after jury awards.

Step 2. According to First et al. (1995), once Malingering Disorder and Factitious Disorder have been ruled out, the evaluator should next consider and rule out issues related to substance use, abuse, and toxicity. The DSM-IV-TR (APA, 2000) defines a substance as a medication, a drug of abuse, or a toxin that usually affects the central nervous system directly. First et al. claimed, "virtually any presentation that is encountered in a mental health setting can be caused by substance use" (p. 2). It is possible to conclude, therefore, that any forensic examination of PTSD should also include specific procedures for deciding if substance use/abuse/toxicity is present, as these conditions might also account for PTSD symptoms.

These two conditions, however, are not necessarily mutually exclusive. Substantial evidence exists in support of the notion that substance abuse and PTSD can be co-morbid conditions (Green, 1995). In addition, outcome research reports (c.f., McFarlane & Yehuda, 1996) indicate that many individuals who have PTSD also demonstrate a poor quality of life that includes the use/abuse of substances, as well as depression and suicide attempts. This being the case, the judicial forum would generally want to know the answer to specific questions, including: (a) did the PTSD developed first and lead to the other problems; (b) were the other problems already in place and only exacerbated by the later development of PTSD; or (c) are the conditions mutually exclusive (Green, 1995)?

Step 3. Third, First et al. (1995) advised that ruling out general medical disorders or making a differential mental health diagnosis when general medical disorders are present is extremely difficult. They have identified four major reasons for this difficulty: (a) some general medical conditions can have the same symptom presentation as many psychiatric disorders; (b) the *initial* presentation of some general medical conditions is often psychiatric in nature; (c) the affiliation between a general medical condition and its psychiatric symptoms may be complex; and (d) individuals are frequently seen by therapists or counselors, in the context of their mental health problems, with little to no recognition of, or consideration for, the potential medical problems with psychiatric consequences.

Several general medical conditions have some of the same symptoms as PTSD. For example, a number of symptoms associated with a mild head injury are similar to those of PTSD, including short-term memory loss, difficulty with concentration, and psychogenic amnesia (Simon, 1995b). Other general medical conditions involve symptoms of anxiety (e.g., endocrine conditions, cardiovascular conditions, respiratory conditions, metabolic conditions, and neurological conditions), which present either initially or as part of a total presentation (APA, 2000). Due to their lack of medical training or lack of familiarity with the medical conditions that should be considered, many clinicians might diagnose PTSD without looking for the medical conditions that might also account for the symptoms. Thus, it is imperative for the forensic examiner to utilize some methodology to rule out any general medical condition that might contribute to a misdiagnosis of PTSD.

Step 4. Once malingering/feigning, substance use/abuse/toxicity, and/or a general medical condition have been ruled out, the forensic examiner can justifiably proceed in diagnosing PTSD. Simon (1995b) has listed five standard questions that every forensic examiner should ask when making a diagnosis of PTSD for court purposes. These questions include: (a) does the alleged PTSD claim actually meet specific clinical criteria for this disorder; (b) is the traumatic stressor that is alleged to have caused the PTSD of sufficient severity to produce this disorder; (c) what is the pre-incident psychiatric history of the claimant; (d) is the diagnosis of PTSD based solely on the subjective reporting of symptoms by the claimant; and (e) what is the claimant's actual level of functional psychiatric impairment?

The phrase "specific clinical criteria" usually refers to the criteria set forth by the DSM-IV-TR (APA, 2000). Using alternative criteria that may be arbitrary or idiosyncratic in nature can leave the forensic examiner vulnerable to a Daubert challenge for failing to use endorsed PTSD standards. In Simon's (1995b) second question, "sufficient severity" refers to the fact that individuals must perceive themselves or another person to be at risk of death or serious bodily harm as the result of a traumatic experience in order to warrant a diagnosis of PTSD (APA, 2000). The answer to this question, therefore, speaks to both an examiner's ability to make an accurate diagnosis of PTSD and to the potential of malingering. In addition, while the third question attempts to identify any previous psychiatric history that could account for the reported symptoms, the fourth question looks for corroboration and consultation to support the claimant's assertions of PTSD symptoms. Finally, the fifth question attempts to obtain a rating of emotional impairment.

It is not uncommon for medical doctors to define the degree of physical impairment that a patient is experiencing in terms of percentages of whole body impairment. For example, a physician might consider an individual who has lost some percentage of mobility in one arm to experience an 18% loss in whole body functioning. Although the American Medical Association's *Guides to the Evaluation of Permanent Impairment* (Cocchiarella & Andersson, 2000) has become the most frequently used source for estimating and rating permanent physical impairment, it presently advises that "there are no precise measures of impairment in mental disorders" (p. 361). In fact, the authors were so adamant about this issue that they included an admonishment they had received from the Committee on Disability and Rehabilitation of the American Psychiatric Association, recommending against the use of percentages to estimate mental impairment when formulating their previous edition of this volume in 1993. As a result, the existing techniques for rating mental impairment do not include percentages. Nevertheless, it has been this author's experience that there are agencies, attorneys, and others who will demand the forensic examiner provide a mental impairment rating using a percentage format.

It is difficult by any standard, however, to state the degree of one's emotional disability, including the symptoms of PTSD, in a percentage format. Although there are methods that some examiners use to accomplish this, Keane (1995) has recommended using scales of social role functioning to determine the extent of one's social and occupational impairment. The present author concurs with this recommendation and suggests that the presently used Global Assessment of Functioning

(GAF) scale (APA, 2000) be replaced with Social and Occupational Functioning Assessment Scale (SOFAS) when determining the Axis V diagnosis of a forensic evaluation for PTSD. The SOFAS format is outlined in Appendix B of the DSM-IV-TR (APA, 2000, pp. 817-818) and provides a standardized, defensible set of ratings to evaluate the emotional disability resulting from a given mental disorder (i.e., PTSD). Although these ratings are minimal in definition, they remain valuable to justify why a specific rating was given and they keep the forensic examiner consistent throughout all forensic examinations.

Simon (1995b) has also proposed an excellent set of five guidelines for conducting a forensic psychiatric examination of PTSD. They are: (a) the use of official diagnostic manuals, professional literature, and current research; (b) the need to assess for multiple stressors and to ensure that the traumatic event is sufficient to meet the diagnostic criteria for PTSD; (c) an examination of the examinee's medical and psychiatric history; (d) not relying on the subjective reporting of the examinee alone and not mixing the forensic examination with treatment; and (e) utilizing standard assessment protocols concurrent with clinical assessment. The use of these five guidelines should help the examiner to successfully survive any Daubert challenge when evaluating claims of PTSD in a forensic setting.

Step 5. The next step is for the examiner to differentiate a diagnosis of PTSD from Adjustment Disorder, Anxiety Disorder Not Otherwise Specified, Other Mental Disorders Resulting from Exposure to a Traumatic Stressor Event, and Acute Stress Disorder. First et al. (1995, p. 170) write that PTSD has a "specific response pattern" while an Adjustment Disorder does not. This specific response pattern can last a lifetime (if left untreated or treated unsuccessfully) and is delineated in the DSM-IV-TR (APA, 2000) by the five major segments of a PTSD diagnosis: actual or threatened death or serious injury, intense fear, re-experiencing symptoms, avoidance symptoms, and arousal symptoms. On the other hand, stress brought on by an Adjustment Disorder is neither patterned nor delineated in the DSM-IV-TR (APA, 2000) and can last for only six months (acute) or as long as the stressor event lasts (chronic). In contrast, PTSD usually lasts long after the stressor event has concluded. Similarly, Acute Stress Disorder has a dissimilar pattern from that of PTSD and involves symptoms that exist for no longer than one month following the conclusion of the traumatic experience.

Other mental disorders that could result from exposure to a traumatic stressor event, mentioned earlier in this article, included generalized anxiety disorder, panic disorder (with and without agoraphobia), depression, dissociative disorders, somatization disorders, the intrusive thoughts of Obsessive-Compulsive Disorder, and any preexisting disorders that the traumatic experience may have only exacerbated. A differential diagnosis can be made between these disorders, however, on the basis of both their duration and the presence or absence of the specific response pattern related to PTSD.

Often, a diagnosis of PTSD cannot be made because the symptom presentation does not meet the full criterion outlined in the DSM-IV-TR (APA, 2000). In such instances, a diagnosis of Anxiety Disorder Not Otherwise Specified is warranted. However, treatment for this condition would be the same as for PTSD. In addition, failure to meet full diagnostic criteria for PTSD does not preclude the examinee from experiencing significant emotional consequences from their exposure to a traumatic event. Such emotional consequences can thus be relevant in a forensic evaluation regardless of whether they meet criteria for a diagnosis of PTSD.

Step 6. Finally, one must establish the boundary of PTSD with no mental disorder. The final concern for the forensic examiner in diagnosing PTSD is to ensure the symptomology being presented is due to PTSD and is not differentiated from a non-problematic state of being (i.e., no mental disorder). That is to say, if the client has symptoms but either (a) is not concerned about them, (b) has no resultant social, occupational, or academic problems, or (c) the symptoms are a result of some developmental consequence, then PTSD cannot be diagnosed. The DSM-IV-TR (APA, 2000) is very clear about symptomology that disrupts one's life in some way as being the only symptomology that can legitimately be diagnosed. First et al. (1995) suggest there is a fine line between the differentiation of one disorder (e.g., PTSD) from another, and clinical judgment is essential.

DATA USED TO SUPPORT OR REFUTE A DIAGNOSIS OF PTSD

The Forensic Examination for Emotional Trauma

Probably the most salient component of a PTSD forensic examination is the Independent Medical Examination (IME) for Emotional Trauma. Although the entire PTSD forensic examination has a number of facets, Litz and Weathers (1994) have asserted that the clinical examination or interview is " the foundation of the PTSD assessment" (p. 20). Further, it is the proposed foundation for gathering all corroborative evidence. The IME for Emotional Trauma includes a clinical interview of the examinee, which is used to determine the notable features of concern. Because the clinical interview is so important, it is recommended that a transcript (usually transcribed by a court reporter) of the clinical interview be made.

One of the major elements of the IME for Emotional Trauma involves taking an examinee's complete history. The present author, clinically trained as a marriage and family therapist, has a decided systemic disposition to history taking. Systems theory dictates that any trauma experienced by one family member affects not only the family system, but also other systems (Harris, 2000). According to this perspective, not only is the family an excellent repository for relevant knowledge and facts about the examinee, but also other systems (e.g., work, school, church, clubs, etc.) with which the examinee is associated. These systems may possess additional information regarding the examinee's symptoms and behaviors. However, from this author's perspective the caveat is that these same systems can, and often do, support malingering. Regardless, the systems bias remains forensically sound.

The history-taking process usually encompasses the following three time periods of an examinee's life: pre-traumatic event, the traumatic event itself, and posttraumatic event. The pre-traumatic event history includes information regarding the examinee's psychiatric, medical, and substance use history, as well as symptoms and behaviors prior to the traumatic event. A history of the traumatic event involves identifying the actual feelings, behaviors, and actions that took place during the traumatic event. The post-traumatic event history includes information regarding an examinee's medical and substance use history, as well as symptoms and behaviors following the traumatic event. All of this information provides a base that will ideally be corroborated in some fashion (e.g., the confirmation of witnesses, statements by family members, statements by others who have knowledge, informally written depositions, formal depositions, etc.). After the IME for Emotional Trauma, it is imperative to examine others who have relevant information that can either confirm or refute the facts offered by the examinee. Due to the potential consequences for the examinee in a forensic setting, whenever possible the examiner should not rely solely on the statements of the examinee to formulate opinions.

Other Components of a PTSD Forensic Examination

A relevant PTSD forensic examination commonly includes (but is not limited to) the previously mentioned IME for Emotional Trauma and the corroborative interview(s). In addition, the following sources of information are also frequently included: (a) clinical assessment(s) for PTSD; (b) document review; (c) a full five axis diagnosis; (d) identification of causal relationships; (e) recommendations for present and/or future treatment (if required); (f) clinical justification/rationale for treatment (if required); (g) reasonable fees for present and/or future treatment (if required); (h) level of emotional impairment and prognosis; and (i) deviations for recognized standards of care. The attorney that engages the forensic services usually determines what is compulsory in any given forensic examination.

According to Cooperstein (1999), a comprehensive assessment for PTSD should address the following prominent issues: (a) the nature and degree of trauma; (b) personality traits and other mental health disorders; (c) the social milieu; (d) the social support network; and (e) the post-trauma model of the world (temporary or permanent). Additionally, the forensic examination should include a mental status inquiry, psychiatric history, a review of the examinee's pre-trauma life, and some evidence of differential diagnosis.

The Identification of Causal Relationships

The identification of causal relationships is probably the most important issue of concern for the legal system. The causal relationship is the factor that makes the traumatic event culpable for a resulting emotional injury. However, most clinicians who took graduate-level statistics courses were taught never to use causality when defining relationships within the probability theory. Instead, clinicians are taught to define these relationships in terms of correlation (e.g., Pearson *r*, Spearman rho, etc.). Such is not the case in forensic examination. The legal system needs to trace the exact line of determination as to who or what was responsible for bringing about another's suffering (i.e., who caused the traumatic event resulting in the victim's PTSD). Forensic examiners must therefore be comfortable discussing such relationships in terms of causality.

Many times, a forensic examiner is asked to make recommendations regarding an examinee's need for present and/or future PTSD treatment. This might include justification for treatment, recommendations for treatment paradigms, suggestions regarding the expense of such treatments, treatment providers, duration of treatment, and the potential outcome of treatment (i.e., prognosis). This kind of information is useful to the triers of fact (i.e., judges and juries) in establishing monetary awards for PTSD.

Forensic Examination of Documents and/or Treatment Records

A common component of a forensic examination involves the review of depositions, records, reports, opinions, testimony, interrogations, and other documents to determine if recognized standards associated with PTSD (usually prevention, assessment, diagnosis, and/or treatment) were employed or violated. Such a forensic review can come from the Plaintiff, the Defense, or as a request of the court. Common documents or records reviewed may include: (a) records and testimony of potential defendants; (b) records and testimony of previous treating psychotherapists; (c) records and testimony of current treating psychotherapists; (d) chronology of significant events; (e) court documents; (f) plaintiff's depositions and answers to interrogatories; and (g) defendant's depositions and answers to interrogatories. In addition, other miscellaneous records or sources of information that are used include: (a) other expert's reports; (b) second-hand records; (c) statements of family members; (d) statements of other relatives; and (e) statements from others who possess relevant knowledge.

The Forensic Examination Report

Under Federal Rule of Civil Procedure 26(2)(B), the forensic expert must prepare and sign a written report that contains the elements listed in Table 2. Babitsky et al. (2000) suggest that failure to adhere to Rule 26(2)(B) could result in the forensic expert's testimony (or findings in any form) being disallowed by the court. However, this being said, a caveat is offered. The forensic examiner is cautioned about writing any report (or draft/notes of same) without the express direction of the attorney contracting for the forensic examination. A forensic examiner does not have confidentiality or privilege regarding the written materials s/he produces as a result of contracted services. As such, all written materials are subject to discovery at any time (during the ongoing litigation or in a future litigation). Discovery is based on the concept that if everyone knows all the evidence that will be presented in a case (including the experts' opinions), the case may be considered fairly (no sur-

TABLE 2. Forensic Report Requirements Under Federal Rule of Civil Procedure 26(2)(B)

- A complete statement of all opinions to be expressed
- The basis and reasons for the opinions
- The data or other information considered
- Any exhibits to be used in summary of the opinions
- Any exhibits to be used as support for the opinions
- The qualifications of the witness
- A list of all publications authored by the witness in the preceding ten years
- The compensation to be paid for the study and testimony
- A listing of any other cases in which the witness has testified as an expert at trial or by deposition within the preceding four years

prises) and potentially settled. Some information may be considered "attorney's work product" (i.e., work in progress that is not usually discoverable until finished), and is thereby protected. See Babitsky et al. for a good description of discovery versus attorney work product.

The opinion(s) proffered by the forensic expert must be based on reliable information, details, and procedures. Usually the opinion is stated in a manner that implies it is "more than 50% likely" or "more likely than not" (Babitsky et al., 2000). In other words, the opinion is based on a reasonable degree of likelihood, not conjecture. For example, a PTSD-oriented opinion might read as follows: "Based on a reasonable degree of therapeutic certainty, Mr. Jones' emotional problems are directly attributable to the automobile crash of August 19, 1999."

IMPORTANT CHARACTERISTICS OF THE EXAMINER

Forensic examiners need to remain constantly aware of the fact that their advocacy is to the finding, the opinion, or the facts gleaned from the examination, rather than to the client or examinee, as it would be during a clinical evaluation. All biases and prejudices must be put aside. Objectivity is hard to achieve, yet it remains the golden chalice of this type of work. The constant striving for objectivity and neutrality is what makes a forensic examination so valuable and crucial in a court of law.

The integrity of the forensic examiner is always at risk and is often attacked in court (as a means to discredit the expert's opinion). Many times, forensic examiners are viewed as "hired guns" that will offer any opinion for the right price. As a result, the PTSD forensic examiner must be able to withstand such scrutiny. Examiners that are most likely to do so and, therefore, are used the most are those who (a) continue to be active in their counseling/therapy practices, providing both assessment and treatment for PTSD; (b) pursue continuing education with respect to both PTSD and forensics; and (c) are consistent with their opinions. Furthermore, the opinions of such examiners regarding similar cases will have typically been upheld in other court proceedings. In other words, the examiner previously has testified regarding a particular issue and the examiner's opinions regarding that issue have been sustained.

CONCLUSION

The diagnosis of posttraumatic stress disorder (PTSD) has truly changed the way emotional damages are awarded in our judicial system. The forensic examination of PTSD is an objective methodology (non-biased and non-prejudicial) that can help establish the critical elements of substantiating PTSD in the examinee.

NOTE

1. See Edwards (1998) for a more detailed description of *Daubert*.

REFERENCES

American Psychiatric Association. (1980). *The diagnostic and statistical manual of mental disorders* (3rd ed.). Washington, DC: Author.

American Psychiatric Association. (1994). *The diagnostic and statistical manual of mental disorders* (4th ed.). Washington, DC: Author.

American Psychiatric Association. (2000). *The diagnostic and statistical manual of mental disorders* (4th ed., text revision). Washington, DC: Author.

Babitsky, S., Mangraviti, J. J., & Todd, C. J. (2000). *The comprehensive forensic services manual: The essential resources for all experts.* Falmouth, MA: SEAK, Inc.

Briere, J. (2001). *DAPS: Detailed Assessment of Posttraumatic Stress Professional Manual.* Odessa, FL: Psychological Assessment Resources, Inc.

Carlson, E. B. (1997). *Trauma assessments: A clinician's guide.* New York: The Guilford Press.

Cocchiarella, L., & Andersson, G. B. (2000). *Guides to the evaluation of permanent impairment* (5th ed.). Washington, DC: AMA Press.

Cooperstein, A. M. (1999). Post-traumatic stress: Consciousness and other correlates in the assessment and treatment of PTSD. *The Forensic Examiner, 8,* 18-24.

Daubert v. Merrell Dow Pharmaceuticals, Inc., 509 U.S. 579 (1993).

Early, E. (1990). Imagined, exaggerated, and malingered post-traumatic stress disorder. In C. L. Meek (Ed.), *Post-traumatic stress disorder: Assessment, differentia diagnosis, and forensic evaluation* (pp. 137-156). Sarasota, FL: Professional Resource Exchange.

Edwards, C. N. (1998). *Responsibilities and dispensations: Behavior, science, & American justice.* Dover, MA: Four Oaks Press.

First, M. B., Frances, A., & Pincus H. A. (1995). *DSM-IV handbook of differential diagnosis.* Washington, DC: American Psychiatric Press.

Frances, A., First, M. B., & Pincus, H. A. (1995). *DSM-IV guidebook.* Washington, DC: American Psychiatric Press.

Goldberg, R. L. (1995). Foreword. In R. I. Simon (Ed.), *Posttraumatic stress disorder: Guidelines for forensic assessment* (p. xiii). Washington, DC: American Psychiatric Press.

Green, B. L. (1995). Recent research findings on the diagnosis of posttraumatic stress disorder: Prevalence, course, comorbidity, and risk. In R. I. Simon (Ed.), *Posttraumatic stress disorder: Guidelines for forensic assessment* (pp. 13-29). Washington, DC: American Psychiatric Press.

Greenfield, D. P. (1999). Psychiatric/psychological evaluations should not be observed or recorded by opposing counsel. *The Forensic Examiner* (January/February), 8.

Harris, C. J. (2002). Traumatic stress in family systems. In M. B. Williams & J. F. Sommer (Eds.), *Clinical competence in the treatment of PTSD* (pp. 261-275). New York: The Haworth Press, Inc.

Keane, T. M. (1995). Guidelines for the forensic psychological assessment of posttraumatic stress disorder claimants. In R. I. Simon (Ed.), *Posttraumatic stress disorder: Guidelines for forensic assessment* (pp. 99-115). Washington, DC: American Psychiatric Press.

Larson, G. A. (Executive Producer). (1976). *Quincy, M.E.* [Television series]. New York: CBS Broadcasting, Inc.

Litz, B. T., & Weathers, F. W. (1994). The diagnosis and assessment of post-traumatic stress disorder in adults. In M. B. Williams & J. F. Sommer (Eds.), *Handbook of post-traumatic therapy* (pp. 19-37). Westport, CT: Greenwood Press.

Matson, Jack V. (1999). *Effective expert witnessing* (3rd ed.). Boca Raton, FL: CRC Press.

McFarlane, A. C., & Yehuda, R. (1996). Resilience, vulnerability, and the course of posttraumatic reactions. In B. A. van der Kolk, A. C. McFarlane, & L. Weisaeth (Eds.), *Traumatic stress: The effects of overwhelming experience on mind, body and society* (pp. 155-181). New York: The Guilford Press.

McKenzie, C. D. (2001). Integrative psychiatry: Prevention & treatment of serious mental and emotional disorders. *Carolina Health & Healing* (Spring Issue).

Modlin, H. C. (1990). Post-traumatic stress disorder: Differential diagnosis. In C. L. Meek (Ed.), *Post-traumatic stress disorder: Assessment, differential diagnosis, and forensic evaluation* (pp. 63-72). Sarasota, FL: Professional Resource Exchange.

Resnick, P. J. (1997). Malingering of posttraumatic disorders. In R. Rogers (Ed.), *Clinical assessment of malingering and deception: Second edition* (pp. 130-152). New York: The Guilford Press.

Simon, R. I. (1995a). *Posttraumatic stress disorder: Guidelines for forensic assessment.* Washington, DC: American Psychiatric Press.

Simon, R. I. (1995b). Toward the development of guidelines in the forensic psychiatric examination of posttraumatic stress disorder claimants. In R. I. Simon (Ed.), *Posttraumatic stress disorder: Guidelines for forensic assessment* (pp. 31-84). Washington, DC: American Psychiatric Press.

Stamm, B. H. (1996). *Measurement of stress, trauma, and adaptation.* Lutherville, MD: Sidran Press.

van der Kolk, B. A., & McFarlane, A. C. (1996). The black hole of trauma. In B. A. van der Kolk, A. C. McFarlane, & L. Weisaeth (Eds.), *Traumatic stress: The effects of overwhelming experience on mind, body, and society* (pp. 3-23). New York: The Guilford Press.

Zuiker, A., Bruckheimer, J., Mendelsohn, C., Donahue, A., Hart, J. C., Littman, J. et al. (Executive Producers). (2000). *CSI* [Television series]. New York: CBS Broadcasting, Inc.

Thought Field Therapy:
Working Through Traumatic Stress
Without the Overwhelming Responses

Robert L. Bray

SUMMARY. The first stage in helping individuals recover from traumatic events requires managing the overwhelming symptoms of reexperiencing, avoidance or numbing, and increased arousal. Thought Field Therapy (TFT) has been demonstrated in a variety of practice settings as a safe and effective technique in this first stage of recovery. It does not require the recounting of the events and does not have any apparent negative side effects. The technique, its development, and relevant research are reviewed. Descriptions of the range of settings in which it can be used, including self-care for therapist, are discussed. Its integration into several practice settings is presented. A common TFT procedure is provided for further exploration by practitioners. *[Article copies available for a fee from The Haworth Document Delivery Service: 1-800-HAWORTH. E-mail address: <docdelivery@haworthpress.com> Website: <http://www.HaworthPress.com> © 2006 by The Haworth Press, Inc. All rights reserved.]*

Address correspondence to Robert L. Bray, 5959 Mission Gorge Road, Suite 106, San Diego, CA 92120 (E-mail: rlbray@rlbray.com).

[Haworth co-indexing entry note]: "Thought Field Therapy: Working Through Traumatic Stress Without the Overwhelming Responses." Bray, Robert L. Co-published simultaneously in *Journal of Aggression, Maltreatment & Trauma* (The Haworth Maltreatment & Trauma Press, an imprint of The Haworth Press, Inc.) Vol. 12, No. 1/2, 2006, pp. 103-123; and: *Trauma Treatment Techniques: Innovative Trends* (ed: Jacqueline Garrick, and Mary Beth Williams) The Haworth Maltreatment & Trauma Press, an imprint of The Haworth Press, Inc., 2006, pp. 103-123. Single or multiple copies of this article are available for a fee from The Haworth Document Delivery Service [1-800-HAWORTH, 9:00 a.m. - 5:00 p.m. (EST). E-mail address: docdelivery@haworthpress.com].

Available online at http://www.haworthpress.com/web/JAMT
doi:10.1300/J146v12n01_06

KEYWORDS. Thought Field Therapy, posttraumatic stress, crisis response, self-care for therapist

As a technique used in Traumatic Stress Response work, Thought Field Therapy (TFT) ends emotional and physical symptoms in a matter of moments, eliminates the overwhelming distress experienced, and in most cases effects permanent change in that stimulus. TFT has applications across the entire range of traumatic stress responses, from mild discomfort sensed somewhere in the background of consciousness to the completely demanding deluge of sensory overload resulting from horrifying life experiences. It works well within grief and bereavement models, brief intervention models of all types, and establishes symptom management necessary for long-term psychotherapy.

When a client is stuck in so much emotional pain that he or she cannot think, act, or even respond, TFT eliminates the overwhelming distress. When a memory or another trigger event related to the past freezes your client, TFT will get him to start thinking, responding, and acting in the ways he wants. When efforts to change the way your client sees herself are frustrated by her fear that the horrible events from her past will happen again, TFT will eliminate the fear and allow her to think of a future with different possible outcomes. By eliminating the overwhelming pain and fear, TFT allows the self-healing mechanisms of the person and the assistance offered by professional intervention to improve their lives.

This article provides the most basic TFT intervention for traumatic stress in a step-by-step protocol. The reader is invited to test for him/herself the validity and power of TFT. The process is safe with no negative side effects. Either the TFT works or it does not work. TFT will not cause harm. TFT does not require the retelling of the events; just think of the event for an instant and then proceed. TFT does not require a belief in its efficacy to work. To investigate for yourself, all that you need is a curious mind and an honest evaluation. The simplest treatment protocol presented here is only one of the many TFT treatment components and focuses on traumatic stress responses; other protocols and elements of TFT are used to relieve other conditions.

Examples of TFT applications for crisis intervention, Acute Distress Disorder, Posttraumatic Stress Disorder (PTSD), Disorders of Extreme Stress Not Otherwise Specified, and self-care for vicarious traumatization are interspersed throughout the article to illustrate the use of TFT in traumatic stress work. These examples of actual clients and experiences are written in the first person to portray more accurately the experience of using TFT with clients.

EXAMPLE 1: SHRINKING THE SHOOTER

In April 2001, an 18-year-old former high school student came onto campus and opened fire with a shotgun. He was in a grassy area between two classroom buildings and was clearly seen by staff, teachers, and students. When he fired several shots into the administration building, a local police officer on campus immediately returned fire. The shooter retreated behind the building and, in a matter of moments, had been wounded and was apprehended by the police officer and a deputy sheriff. When school resumed three days later, I provided critical incident stress management with the staff and students in one of those classrooms. After working with the students in a group format, I worked one-on-one with an adult who was clearly having trouble with his emotions as he talked about his experience of the events. He described his worst memory/experience as seeing the shooter firing his weapon. He had been in the shooter's clear line of sight as he moved students out a back door into another classroom. His identified Subjective Unit of Distress (SUD) was eight on a ten-point scale (very upset) as he began to tap with his fingertips on treatment points on his body. After the first round of tapping (the technique is described later in this article), he was calmer and reported that the picture in his mind was changing. As we started, he said that the shooter appeared to be taller than the buildings, but as we tapped, the shooter started to shrink. By the time we completed the third round of tapping, he rated his SUD as one and reported that the shooter was back to normal size. We both then returned to our duties with the students. At the end of the day, his memory of the shooting included a very normal sized assailant and he was able to talk about the events with practically no effort. This example of crisis intervention was with someone who was clearly overwhelmed and upset, but still functioning. Some of the best work with TFT occurs before the symptoms have developed into impairments to functioning. This intervention took less than five minutes and was done in the middle of other work.

WHAT IS THOUGHT FIELD THERAPY?

In this article, TFT refers to Callahan Techniques® Thought Field Therapy (CTTFT).[1] Over the last 25 years, Roger Callahan, PhD, has been the driving force in the development and refinement of this revolutionary practice. In simple terms, it appears that the control mechanism of the emotions and all physiology of a person is accessible through the energy systems of acupuncture. By simulating meridian treatment points (sites where needles or pressure are applied in Chinese medicine), TFT makes subtle changes in this control mechanism. TFT activates these points by having the client tap on the points with their fingertips. The order of tapping provides information to change the coding in the control mechanism that prompts the negative emotions. By making subtle changes in the coding on the control mechanism through the meridian system, there are rapid and blatantly discernable changes in the emotional and physiological systems of the person. The formal definition of TFT is as follows:

> Thought Field Therapy is a treatment for psychological disturbances which provides a code, that, when applied to a psychological problem the person is focusing on, will eliminate the perturbations in the thought field, the fundamental cause of all negative emotions. This code is elicited through TFT's causal diagnostic procedure, through which the TFT algorithms were developed. (Callahan & Trubo, 2001, p. 4)

Dr. Callahan has written much on the application, theory, and other aspects of TFT. The best source for a comprehensive discussion of the current TFT theory is found in Dr. Callahan's books (Callahan & Callahan, 2000; Callahan & Trubo, 2001). A full discussion on TFT theory is beyond the scope of this article and is not required at this time. Just as a belief in TFT's efficacy in not necessary for TFT to work, a full understanding of the mechanism of action is not necessary for a practitioner be successful in the application of TFT.

Over five thousand people have completed TFT workshops and thousands more have used it. Within the psychological and counseling professions, TFT has been used effectively to treat a broad range of conditions. For example, one study involved 714 patients from behavioral medicine services and behavioral health services who were treated with TFT for 31 categories of problems or symptoms (Sakai et al., 2001). In all, 1,594 applications showed statistical significance for in-session reductions in self-reported distress. Conditions treated included trichotillomania, nicotine and alcohol cravings, Obsessive-Compulsive Disorder, depression, chronic pain, and a variety of stress-related conditions. Often, TFT will provide relief when traditional psychological approaches have failed. For example, James Schaefer (2002) describes his personal struggles with Obsessive-Compulsive Disorder and anxiety and how these problems were corrected using TFT. After more than 20 years of trying other forms of treatment with no lasting success, TFT treatments brought him to a functional lifestyle.

Beyond psychological services, TFT is now used in many other professional settings, such as physical medicine where it is been used to improve a number of conditions. Most notably, TFT will improve heart rate variability (HRV). Established by basic research to be a stable and placebo-free measure, HRV is considered as the best predictor of mortality after a cardiac event (Tsuji et al., 1996). Research has demonstrated that TFT can improve HRV (Callahan, 2001a, 2001b; Pignotti & Bray, 2000; Pignotti & Steinberg, 2001). Nursing (Cooper, 2001), psychiatry, chiropractic medicine, education, religion, sports psychology, acupuncture, physical therapy, and many other healing settings are using TFT, as reported by practitioners in the Callahan Techniques newsletter, *The Thought Field*.

TFT is one of the most effective means of controlling the symptoms of traumatic stress in a matter of moments, and, in most cases, the change with that particular stimulus is permanent (Carbonell & Figley, 1999; Folkes, 2002; Edwards, 1998; Johnson, Shala, Sejdijaj, Odell, & Dabishevci, 2001). In some cases, all the symptoms related to a critical incident may be resolved in one treatment sequence. It is also possible that each aspect of a memory or other related triggers provoking the negative responses may need to be addressed as they arise one at a time. If that happens, TFT can be repeated for that new trigger. TFT provides for quick and complete symptom elimination rather than "management." This allows the therapy to focus on other aspects of traumatic stress recovery work, such as re-working the trauma or integrating the trauma as it is needed. Indeed, TFT has been so effective in Kosovo that it has been adopted on a national level by the Surgeon General of Kosovo. In a letter dated January 11, 2001, to Dr. Callahan from Dr. Shkelzen Syla, Chief of Staff of the Medical Battalion with authority for all medical decisions in Kosovo, it was announced that a national program using TFT has been ordered to treat PTSD (Syla, 2001).

EXAMPLE TWO: SEXUAL ASSAULT

Jean was referred by the local prosecutor's office to help her prepare for a preliminary hearing for the man who assaulted her. As session began, she was unable to do anything other than cry as she began to respond to the question, "What happened?" At my direction, she began TFT to help her reduce her upset and help her talk. In less than three minutes, she was able to tell me what happened. As she described the events, she again became upset to the point that she had to stop talking. She was able to report that this upset had to do with the anger and rage she was feeling as she remembered what had happened, a different focus than when she started the session. During the first tapping sequence, she was thinking about how much pain she had felt when she was assaulted. The second tapping sequence was for the anger and rage. She then finished telling the story of the assault.

As she talked about why she was in my office, she became overwhelmed at the thought of having to be in the same room as the perpetrator during the hearing. She then tapped for the associated anxiety. Once she was able to visualize herself testifying, her upset returned as she saw her husband and parents in the courtroom. She acknowledged that her feeling of guilt for putting her loved ones through the hearing was unreasonable and knew she had done nothing wrong. Yet, she could not tolerate the feeling that she was hurting people she loved. Within her family culture, it was not acceptable for her to ask them to not attend court to support her. Next, we tapped for this irrational guilt.

Upon finishing our session, Jean reported that she knew what she had to do to prepare for the court appearance the next day. She decided she would go home and tell her husband and her parents what had happened to her because she wanted them to hear the facts from her in a safe place before they heard it in open court. Jean did not request further assistance. Once she had managed her overwhelming feelings, Jean was able to make sense out of what happened to her and what it meant in her life using her natural support systems. Before she left, she was given a written tapping pattern to use if the feelings became overwhelming again.

Jean's case is a good example of how an overwhelming thought or memory was treated with TFT. After each tapping sequence, it became possible to think about what had happened and what will happen in a new way. In a new thought, there may be another layer of overwhelming emotions. In this example, TFT was used to eliminate each layer as it occurred.

WHAT TFT IS NOT

TFT does not directly change values, beliefs, knowledge, or aesthetics. These are fundamentally cognitive functions and are the result of complex processes in the mind. Value and belief systems are extensive and form over years during the development of the person. There are no demonstrations of TFT changing a person's belief or value structure by tapping. After tapping, persons do not have access to factual information not already held. However, when TFT is used to reduce stress and anxiety there is improved performance on intellectual tasks, such as reading or learning (Blaich, 1988). Increased stress impedes cognitive functioning in a variety of ways. By reducing these stress responses and/or eliminating other disturbances, a person's functioning will improve, thereby accounting for noticeably enhanced performance on familiar tasks that may appear to be a change in intelligence. The same, perhaps, is true for memory. By removing barriers such as unneeded fear or anxiety, it is possible to improve focus and be capable of providing more detailed reports. Memory is mastered more quickly, and access to memories is increased when the fear and pain is reduced or eliminated.

TFT does not change reality. TFT does not divorce people from fundamental human processes. We will experience loss and integrate it into our being as it fits our nature, no matter what we do. We will grieve and experience bereavement even when we have eliminated the overwhelming emotions or recurrent intrusive images.

Since TFT does not directly change values or beliefs, it is not possible to tap away personality disorders. Personality disorders are descriptions of sets of individual traits developed over years that result in dysfunctional coping and relationship patterns. They are not the result of one event, tendency, or characteristic. Values, beliefs, knowledge, and aesthetics concerning oneself impact the development and maintenance of personality. In the same ways that TFT may improve cognitive functions, TFT can ease and speed personality change. TFT makes reconsidering or changing personality patterns much less stressful. However, it is not possible to "tap in a trait."

Changing lifelong patterns requires conscious repeated efforts in new thinking and behavior. If these new thoughts and behaviors trigger overwhelming upset, it is unlikely the person will practice and incorporate these new thoughts and behaviors. TFT can help in this process of change by removing the overwhelming upset. For example, stating a positive self-affirmation can be the first step to changing negative self-talk, but if a person becomes overwhelmed making such a statement because of prior conditioning, no cognitive reframing occurs. By eliminating the upset, TFT makes it possible to change self-talk quickly.

The work of making cognitive and behavioral change is accelerated with TFT.

Those who are trained in Eye Movement Desensitization and Reprocessing (EMDR) and TFT understand that they are completely different interventions and approaches. EMDR sometimes has the client mentally track tapping on alternating palms of the hands as part of their protocol to make bilateral shifts in the brain. This tapping is not related to TFT in any way. EMDR is primarily a cognitive technique and an informational processing model with a physiological component (Shapiro, 1995). TFT is based in a completely different paradigm and is not a cognitive technique.

EXAMPLE THREE:
STUCK WITH THE SYMBOL:
WHEN OTHER TAPPING DOES NOT WORK

At a conference workshop on self-care, I asked for a volunteer to demonstrate TFT. A woman who had already shared some of her history came forward. She was a well-trained professional with extensive experience in traumatic stress recovery work in many roles. Two years earlier, she had coordinated an extensive response to multiple-line-of-duty deaths. She clearly had done a very good job in providing for the survivors, families, employees, responders, and her own staff. She had even sought out a therapist to help her work through her own responses to this once-in-a-lifetime set of circumstances. The current problem was that, years after the event, she still encountered symbolic triggers in her daily life that would stimulate overwhelming emotional responses. Her responses were wearing on her in a chronic way. She had stopped seeing her therapist after a year because there had been little improvement in managing the symbolic triggers. While she was still functional, she acknowledged she was at high risk for both burnout or compassion fatigue. When I suggested we try some tapping to relieve the overwhelming feelings associated with these symbolic triggers, she stated that she was familiar with tapping, as her therapist had used it with her. However, she reported that it had not worked on this issue. Her description of the tapping patterns and procedures used made it clear her therapist had not used current TFT, even though it had some TFT components. Using the TFT trauma protocol, she was able to end her emotional upset in a matter of moments. Several other professionals in the workshop verified an observable change in her physical appearance, as well as in her subsequent discussions of the event and the symbol. The next day, she reported that her fiancée said that for the first time, he could see a physical change in her when she discussed these issues. This example illustrates that it is imperative to use the correct tapping protocol to achieve the predicted results.

THE EVOLUTION OF TFT

It is important to review the rigorous methods used to develop TFT if one is to make sense of this fast and effective new approach. Without this frame of reference, it is all too easy to dismiss TFT. TFT is not magic, nor was it revealed in a moment of cosmic attunement. Dr. Callahan was a radio operator and aerial gunner on a B-24 bomber in WWII before obtaining his PhD in clinical psychology from Syracuse University in 1955. He worked for years as a therapist, educator, and researcher before his first experiences with what lead to TFT. From the beginning of his career, his inquisitive mind and his commitment to finding ways to help individuals with anxiety and other debilitating disorders motivated him to explore approaches to helping that were outside the mainstream. He evaluated many techniques on their own merits; as a result, he became a fellow in clinical hypnosis in the early 1950s. He was also a trainer for Albert Ellis and established the first Rational Emotive Therapy Center outside of New York. In addition, he was an author in the first double blind study of psychiatric medications (Callahan, Graham, & Rosenblum, 1958). His list of accomplishments and affiliations in his first fifty years of life before TFT is impressive.

About twenty-five years ago, Dr. Callahan was introduced to muscle testing while in private practice treating anxiety disorders. Intrigued, he took formal training in Applied Kinesiology and began to experiment with applications of this chiropractic approach for healing in the psychological realm. Dr. Callahan was the first person to use muscle testing to develop a reliable and valid way to identify the fundamental source of a psychological problem and the treatments needed to dramatically help and eliminate psychological problems. This led to finding specific treatments for a large number of psychological problems including depression, phobias, anxiety, panic, guilt, and trauma. Each advancement in TFT techniques began as an experiment in making a positive change in an individual. Careful examination and experimentation led to expanded diagnostic and treatment protocols that formed the basis of Causal Diagnosis. Causal Diagnosis is what makes TFT different from other psychological approaches. As a result of making positive change in people, TFT theory was developed as a way to make sense of the reality revealed by these successful treatments. Inductive reasoning underlines all of TFT development (Callahan & Callahan, 2000).

One of the most significant ways in which TFT differs from other approaches is that treatment is precise and specific; there is no guesswork. In all other psychological approaches, the therapist gathers the history and current signs and symptoms to place the person's condition in a category of disorder. Then, based on that best assessment, the treatment generally used for that category occurs. With TFT Causal Diagnosis, the person's specific needs and problems are addressed. The relationship between emotional states and meridian treatment points is specific and precise, as demonstrated with muscle testing. The required treatment is also specific and precise. After observing thousands of cases using Causal Diagnostic, Dr. Callahan identified recurring patterns that provided the basis for the standard patterns of treatments. These patterns are extremely effective in resolving the overwhelming states, and are called TFT Algorithms. Experiences of TFT trained interventionists of all professional types generally find that the algorithms are about 80% effective in eliminating all traumatic stress symptoms.

When one algorithm does not work to eliminate the distress, other algorithms may. Within an hour session, a professional trained at the Algorithm Level can easily explore all the possible algorithms and other standard components of TFT to find an algorithm that works or identify a need for more advanced Causal Diagnosis. A practitioner trained in Causal Diagnosis is able to discern the exact tapping sequence to help the client. At this level, most trauma survivors will learn how to cope with their symptoms. Practitioners trained in Causal Diagnosis find that 3-5% of the general population needs to make additional changes in some aspects of their food choices or other lifestyle elements to achieve long-term cures. These changes can be identified by Causal Diagnostics and are particular to the individual. There are no general prohibitions regarding foods or lifestyle in TFT. The full explanation of the necessity for these changes is well developed elsewhere (Callahan & Callahan, 2000) and it is sufficient for the novice TFT practitioner to be aware of expected results and additional elements when needed.

Once the immediate symptoms are relieved, it then becomes possible to identify and address other issues. Bereavement, family of origin issues, previous traumas, dysfunctional coping patterns, substance abuse, self-esteem, problem solving and decision-making, and/or relationships are some of the areas to address as necessary. For some clients, once their primary symptoms are eliminated, they can take on other issues in their lives. Regardless of the psychotherapeutic approach used, TFT allows quicker and more focused work (Callahan & Callahan, 1997; Carbonell & Figley, 1999; Wade, 1990).

EXAMPLE FOUR: JUST GIVING THE GUY A CHANCE

Joe was referred by his Employee Assistance Program about two months after completing a 12-week cognitive therapy outpatient treatment program for depression. While the treatment had been successful in greatly reducing the suicidal risk for this 50-year-old firefighter, he was still miserable and knew he could again slip back to taking out his gun. He, also, now knew that he was suffering from PTSD, as a result of over 25 years in the fire service.

The problem, as he related it, started after working for 15 years in a low income, diverse neighborhood. His duties included daily medical runs for domestic violence, gang-related shootings, criminal victimization, and responding to calls related to all the other suffering that comes from extreme poverty. As a young white firefighter, he welcomed the opportunity to make a difference in people's lives and rose quickly to leadership roles. Then one day after years of service his truck responded to the shooting death of a police officer, and he felt the risk he and the crew were facing. After subsequent similar events, he lost any sense of security. No longer did he feel as if the people he served welcomed his presence. Increasingly, he felt that everyone was a threat.

After the transfer to a quiet duty station, he lost interest in his job and just "put in his time." However, the feeling of being unsafe did not go away. Joe became more unhappy and afraid. He started carrying a gun everywhere he went, and answered the door only when he had his gun. He also worried constantly about the safety of his wife and sons. He stopped going out in public with them because he was afraid of what he would have to do to protect them. He was no longer comfortable when he was alone in public places. When he perceived himself to be in a crowd, his anxiety went up. When the crowd appeared to focus on him, his fear overtook him and he had to get out or somehow take control, yet he was afraid of what he might do to take that control.

He could not explain his feelings or behavior to his wife. When he put the gun to his head and talked about shooting himself, his wife demanded he seek help. The initial help he received taught him how to express some of what he was feeling and how to make sense out of those feelings. Coupled with medication, this brought some relief. Joe felt less "crazy" and gave up carrying the gun. Yet, he was still very unhappy. He was not sleeping well, and he was still afraid for his family in public places and could not go out with them. The PTSD, recognized as a co-morbid condition in the depression treatment, became the primary concern as he more fully disclosed many of his symptoms and details of his exposures.

Within three sessions, using TFT to resolve the PTSD symptoms, Joe reported a lifting of the depression. It was not difficult to convince him that he needed to continue to see me: he was impressed that after our first session, he was able to lay to rest haunting incidents that had occurred twenty years earlier.

As soon as he learned that he could remember what had happened to him and feel the emotions without getting overwhelmed, Joe started talking about all the critical incidents in his career. He shared the stressors from the community and from the department. When he felt his upset as he told the stories, we tapped, and he then shared more. For the first time in his life, he felt safe with himself and with another human being. Very quickly, he began to address his fears about being in public and within a few weeks, he was able to go out by himself. He gained confidence that it was safe "out there" as he took the time to test, step-by-step, how it felt to move back into the world. Within four months, he was comfortable going out by himself or with his family.

Sessions using TFT now focused on other traumatic stress situations in work and what had happened to him as a child. Primarily, he had been emotionally neglected and abused, with interspersed incidents of physical violence beginning at about age eight. This early trauma was the basis of problems with his current family. TFT allowed him to manage the very uncomfortable feelings that accompanied looking at his family of origin, and allowed him to recognize and understand the power of these early events in shaping his self-identity and his relationship patterns. For the first time in his life, he felt he had a chance to get something he wanted. He was not clear yet about what that was, but there was a sense he could get it.

Over the next six months, he came to sessions once or twice a month when he needed to talk about his feelings or his plans. His family of origin work was greatly accelerated by the use of TFT. He gained insight into his behavior and his coping patterns. His mother was dead and his father unknown to him until very late in his life. After about a year of work, he knew how to tap for himself when the feelings started to become upsetting, and he could make sense of his behavior, so he stopped sessions. He no longer had to wait until feeling completely overwhelmed and dysfunctional to help himself or to ask for help. He knew his limitations in relationships and promised to come back when he decided to get serious about a relationship again.

When he started with me, Joe's condition was very serious and he was still very much at risk. His abuse as a child and the lack of fulfillment of his basic needs in his development was substantial. In less than a year, he accomplished what would have taken years before TFT. As I was writing this article, he called and requested a session for himself and his wife. They are trying again to reconcile. He had kept his promise to seek more help before getting into a serious relationship. Furthermore, tapping is a big part of what allows him to manage his feelings about himself around his wife.

VERIFYING TFT'S EFFECTIVENESS

In TFT, the most important measure of clinical change comes from the person making the changes (i.e., the patient's experience determines the effectiveness of the treatment). Saying that a procedure works just because the theory predicates change, or the clinician has had success with a particular treatment before, or a patient hopes that change has occurred, is meaningless unless the change is substantiated in reality. In TFT, people use a one to ten scale to describe their Subjective Units of Distress (SUD) as they progress through the protocols. Standardized self-report scales have proven to be valid and reliable evidence of the changes in feelings and behaviors. SUD scales avoid confusion about when change is occurring. With each TFT algorithm intervention, the person's SUD report determines the next action.

Clinical observation of facial expressions, posture, eye contact, other body language, skin color, respiration rates, levels of motor activity, vocal tone, and other items found in a standard mental health assessment provide another check on the clients condition pre- and post- TFT. Assessment of cognitive function, such as clarity of thought, expression of ideas, ability to take in new information, acceptance of reframing of events, and access to and mastery of memory provide windows into the change that happens with TFT. Changes in behavior are often seen within sessions after using TFT; for example, a client's engaging with a spouse or family member, addressing subjects never before addressed, or letting go of an issue are powerful demonstrations of TFT. Also, changes in behavior outside of sessions (e.g., stopping self-destructive behavior or doing what was precluded by phobic responses) are for clinicians the acid tests of change.

These direct observations of the impact of TFT do not require special equipment. Other ways of verifying the changes made by TFT are available with additional tools. Changes in the physical body as measured by heart rate, temperature, blood sugar levels, blood pressure, and heart rate variability (HRV) have substantiated TFT's powerful impact (Callahan, 2001a, 2001b; Pignotti & Bray, 2001; Pignotti & Steinberg, 2002). As discussed earlier, HRV sets TFT apart from other therapies. Originally, a cardiac diagnostic tool, HRV has been used as a measure in hundreds of studies. There are over 2000 journal articles, chapters, or books written on HRV over the last 35 years (Huikuri, Makikallio, Airaksinen, Mitrani, Castellanos, & Myerburg, 1999). This placebo-free measure of change has been recently used in studies on PTSD (Cohen et al., 1998) and anxiety (Kawachi, Sparrow, Vokonas, & Weiss, 1995). No matter how the change is measured, TFT produces improvements that can be seen both by the client and the practitioner.

To experience TFT yourself, use the protocol provided in Appendix A, which provides a sense of how TFT changes the subjective response to traumatic memories. As with all TFT, it will either help to reduce the SUD related to the memory or it will do nothing. It will not make it worse and you can continue to use any other coping technique available to you. Focus on a memory of an event in the past that evokes some discomfort. Something that will be rated at about a six on the ten-point scale is all that is required. Those already trained in TFT will recognize the protocol as the standard Complex Trauma with anger and guilt algorithm, with corrections for psychological reversal at the beginning. While this is not a standard Algorithm taught in approved workshops, it provides the untrained person an excellent success rate. Standard algorithms are shorter and more precise in their application.

TFT IN TRAUMATIC STRESS WORK

With TFT, traumatic stress response symptoms are most often resolved quickly and do not return. However, it is not unusual for the person to feel some upset if he/she thinks of another aspect of the event or recalls a different memory associated with the event. As the person clears away the overwhelming distress associated with one memory, he often has an awareness of a distress related to the new thoughts or memories. The rule is to use TFT on each disturbance as it appears. Often treating one aspect of a traumatic event generalizes to the whole event and no other treatment for overwhelming emotions is necessary. Until a therapist receives additional training, it is best to use the extended trauma protocol with clients as a self-help technique. When TFT works, the therapist can give clients a copy of the protocol to use later if they need it.

Using TFT in Crisis Intervention

An interventionist may use the TFT trauma protocol at the scene of a crisis or immediately after to help the person recover functioning. When someone has just directly witnessed a life-threatening event or an event that has impacted a loved one and the person is visibly upset, you do not ask for a SUD. Assume it to be a 10 and have the person mirror tapping the Extended Trauma Protocol. As the person settles down, apply other TFT algorithms and other crisis intervention steps as required or appropriate. After the safety of the person is ensured, restoring functioning is the next step in crisis intervention. TFT helps the person by reducing the overwhelming emotional responses allowing the helper to assist in moving the client to the next steps of the crisis intervention model being used.

TFT is unparalleled in its effectiveness to resolve Acute Stress Disorder symptoms occurring 3 to 30 days after the event. As distress associated with telling the story arises, use the appropriate algorithm to eliminate that distress. When the person can tell the whole story, or can think through the whole story with appropriate (not overwhelming) affect, other concerns about the changes that have occurred as a result of the traumatic events may need to be addressed. For example, after the sudden death of a loved one, more than a one-time TFT session is often required, as there are usually many facets involved. Refer a client to any needed specialist to assist in making life changes. In fact, many grief specialists and spiritual counselors have received training in TFT.

TFT may be used to resolve Posttraumatic Stress Disorder symptoms as they present. Getting to the thought field that needs attention is generally not an issue. The core of the problem is the on-going overwhelming thoughts, sensations, emotions, and memories associated with the events that are beyond the person's control. The person often develops avoidant or addictive behaviors to cope with these symptoms. When there is overwhelming depression, rage, addiction, or pain related to the original trauma, the therapist may need to address these more complex problems/symptoms with a variety of algorithms or with Causal Diagnostic treatments.

Complex and Complicated Disorders of Extreme Stress, the result of many years of overwhelming physical, emotional, or sexual abuse as well as exposure to violence (both threatened and actual) over extended periods of time, can cause destruction of core functions and/or development of extreme coping mechanisms. It is important to use caution while assisting these individuals in managing the overwhelming distress. Respect personal limitations in both TFT treatment and traumatic stress recovery knowledge and skills. If a client changes thought fields at rapid rates, does not slow down, is triggered into a more excited state, or shuts down as they discuss their problems, ensure safety before continuing any treatment.

Self-Care with TFT

When a therapist has heard a story that touches him or her in a way that triggers his or her own experiences, or when a story is too overwhelming, use of the extended trauma protocol or other TFT removes the overwhelming distress and allows the therapist to process a day's work on his/her own. The best self-care for providers comes with competence. If you know what you are doing and can do it well, you have much less chance of hurting others or yourself. Knowing the TFT algorithm for trauma does not make a therapist a competent trauma recovery specialist. The Association of Traumatic Stress Specialist (ATSS) requires training in specific knowledge areas and extensive experience to meet certification criteria for that designation. It is the practitioner's responsibility to have the assessment skills and knowledge to assure that survivors get appropriate help. It is also the practitioner's responsibility to know his or her own limits and capacities to manage the stress of continual exposure to vicarious trauma that is inevitable when experiencing secondarily the horror of critical incidents. The final examples of TFT applications presented here demonstrate the value of TFT in self-care for the therapist doing traumatic stress recovery work.

EXAMPLE FIVE: ENGAGING CLIENTS FEARLESSLY

A client in her 40s once shared an experience that happened to her at about age eight. The level of violence and pain that she had suffered was horrible. She had been sexually, physically, and emotionally brutalized while being forced to watch and participate in similar assaults on others. At some point in the telling of her story, I began to cry, which was not unusual behavior (my rule is: if I will laugh with a client, I will cry with them). However, in this situation my own upset continued to increase as the details of her horrific suffering became too much and I was no longer able to listen. I stopped her recounting the events and treated myself with TFT. Once I had reduced my own upset from this vicarious traumatization, she continued to tell the rest of the details of this event. TFT then helped her with her overwhelming feelings. I was also able to help her by being a witness to the violence she experienced and guide her in making sense of these events and her life.

In the past, before I learned TFT, I would have stopped her from telling me that story. I know that even as skilled and committed as I am to helping others, I would have found a reason to avoid these powerful feelings and protect myself. My excuse may have been that it was too much for *her* to continue. Alternatively, I might have suggested she process these events piece by piece before going on. Through my emotional responses, she may have gotten the message that she was not permitted to hurt me with this story and stopped telling it to me. Thanks to TFT, we continued to the end.

The big payoff for the client came the next week. When I asked, "What stuck with you from the previous session?" she replied, "That in all my life, it was the first time anyone had ever cried about what happened to me as a child." This meant a great deal to her and to me. Our professional relationship has continued to grow. She now trusts that it is safe for her to share her experiences, a first for her in several ways. It is the first time she has been safe enough in a relationship with another person, a man, and/or an authority figure to reveal her story. She knows she does not have to take care of the therapist and that the therapist will be there to help her.

A FINAL EXAMPLE:
STAYING AVAILABLE TO HEAL OURSELVES
AND HELP OTHERS

The speed with which TFT relieves traumatic stress symptoms under any conditions is impressive, and the role of the interventionist is minimal as long as the correct sequence is tapped. At the worst moment of my life, I offered TFT to someone in need. I was attending a memorial service for Trey, an eleven-year-old boy, who had died a week earlier. He was the son of my and my wife's oldest and dearest friends. Trey was at a birthday party for a friend when a strong wind broke a large redwood tree branch that fell on him as he was running by, causing a head injury that left him unconscious. As his mother put it, this was a blameless event. Although EMS arrived in a timely manner and Trey was life-flighted to the hospital, they could not save him. Seven days later, about five hundred people attended the memorial service at a junior high school. Before the service, his mother greeted friends and family. As she hugged a woman, she mouthed the words "help her" to me. I was an emotional wreck. When the woman stepped back, I saw she was in uniform. She was the first EMT on scene and was having a very hard time coping. I identified myself as an International Critical Incident Stress Foundation approved instructor for critical incident stress debriefing and a Certified Trauma Specialist. The woman explained that although she had been to a debriefing, she was unable to get the picture of Trey out of her mind for the last week. On a one to ten scale, the picture in her mind was vivid, disturbing, and a level ten. In the middle of this very crowded room, I led her through one extended trauma algorithm, after which she reported the picture gone. I had treated myself with TFT many times throughout the week. Without it, I would not have been available for that EMT or friends. TFT does not change reality nor interfere with grieving; the loss of Trey continues to be painful. However, TFT gives us a way to keep functional and available for our own healing and for helping others.

CONCLUSION

Only through personal investigation and practice is it possible to appreciate fully the extraordinary help available for therapist and clients with TFT. Being fully trained in TFT requires reading several books on TFT and related subjects, studying audiotapes and videotapes, reading manuals, attending training workshops, and practicing to gain experience. More information about advanced training is available through the Association for Thought Field Therapy (ATFT) or Callahan Techniques Web sites (www.atft.org or www.tftrx.com).

NOTE

1. All articles and studies cited have used CTTFT. All training discussed is CTTFT and approved by the Association for Thought Field Therapy (ATFT). Since making his first foundational discoveries, many of Dr. Callahan's trainees and others have taken parts of his diagnostic and treatment protocols and have made changes and/or renamed

the processes. These derivations of Dr. Callahan's work have maintained some elements, modified some elements, and added a variety of elements. They are related to Dr. Callahan's work and are recognizable in that they use tapping or other stimulation of meridian treatment points in sequence, have a nine gamut series (see Appendix), often employ muscle testing, and/or refer to Dr. Callahan's discoveries. To the extent that these other approaches use TFT elements appropriately, they can be effective. However, they are not the most current or most efficient applications of TFT and should be considered lay applications with limited capacities to eliminate more serious conditions.

REFERENCES

Association for Thought Field Therapy. (2003). *Algorithm level workshop manual.* Indian Wells, CA: Association for Thought Field Therapy

Blaich, R. (1988, Winter). Applied kinesiology and human performance. *Selected papers of the International College of Applied Kinesiology, 1-15.*

Callahan, R. (2001a). The impact of Thought Field Therapy on heart rate variability. *Journal of Clinical Psychology, 57,* 1153.

Callahan, R. (2001b). Raising and lowering of heart rate variability: Some clinical findings of Thought Field Therapy. *Journal of Clinical Psychology, 57,* 1175.

Callahan, R., & Callahan, J. (1997). Thought Field Therapy: Aiding the bereavement process. In C. Figley, B. E. Bride, & N. Mazza (Eds.), *Death and trauma: The traumatology of grieving* (pp. 246-266). Washington: Taylor and Francis

Callahan, R., & Callahan, J. (2000). *Stop the nightmare of trauma.* Chapel Hill, NC: Professional Press

Callahan, R., Graham, B., & Rosenblum, S. (1958). Placebo controlled study of reserpine in maladjusted retarded children. *American Medical Association Journal of Diseases of Children, 96,* 690-695.

Callahan, R., & Trubo, R. (2001) *Tapping the healer within.* New York: Contemporary/McGraw-Hill.

Carbonell, J. L., & Figley, C. (1999). A systematic clinical demonstration of promising PTSD treatment approaches. *Electronic Journal of Traumatology, 5*(1), Article 4 [On-line].

Cohen, H., Kotler, M., Matar, M., Kaplan, Z., Loewenthal, U., Miodownik, H., & Cassuto, Y. (1998). Analysis of heart rate variability in posttraumatic stress disorder patients in response to a trauma-related reminder. *Biological Psychiatry, 44,* 1054-1059.

Cooper, J. (2001). Thought Field Therapy. *Complementary Therapies in Nursing and Midwifery, 7*(3), 162-165.

Edwards, J. (1998). The right place at the right time: Nairobi embassy bombing. *The Thought Field, 4*(3), 1-2.

Folkes, C. (2002). Thought Field Therapy and trauma recovery. *International Journal of Emergency Mental Health, 4*(2), 99-103.

Huikuri, H., Makikallio, T., Airaksinen, K., Mitrani, R., Castellanos, A., & Myerburg, R. (1999). Measurement of heart rate variability: A clinical tool or a research toy? *Journal of the American College of Cardiology, 34*(7), 1878-1883.

Johnson, C., Shala, M., Sejdijaj, X., Odell, R., & Dabishevci, D. (2001). Thought Field Therapy–Soothing the bad moments of Kosovo. *Journal of Clinical Psychology, 57,* 1237-1240.

Kawachi, I., Sparrow, D., Vokonas, P., & Weiss, S. (1995). Decreased heart rate variability in men with phobic anxiety (data from the Normative Aging Study). *American Journal of Cardiology, 75*(14), 882-885.

Pignotti, M., & Bray, R. (2000, November). *Heart rate variability in verifying treatment efficacy of Thought Field Therapy.* Poster session presented at the International Society for Traumatic Stress Studies Annual Meeting. San Antonio, TX.

Pignotti, M., & Steinberg, M. (2001). Heart rate variability as an outcome measure for Thought Field Therapy in clinical practice. *Journal of Clinical Psychology, 57*(10) 1193-1206.

Sakai, C., Paperny, D., Mathews, M., Tanida, G., Boyd, G., Simons, A., Yamamoto, C., Mau, C., Nutter, L. (2001). Thought Field Therapy clinical applications: Utilization in an HMO in behavioral medicine and behavioral health services. *Journal of Clinical Psychology, 57*(10), 1215-1227.

Schaefer, J. (2002). *The pretzel man: A true story of phobias and back problems.* Bloomington, IN: 1st Books.

Shapiro, F. (1995). *Eye movement desensitization and reprocessing: Basic protocols, principles, and procedures.* New York: Guilford

Syla, S. (2001). Letter from Dr. Shkelzen Syla to Dr. Roger Callahan. Retrieved March 21, 2004 from, http://www.thoughtfieldtherapy.net/kosova.html

Tsuji, H., Larson, M. G., Vanditti, F. J., Manders, E. S., Evans, J. C., Feldman, C. L., & Levey, D. (1996). Impact of reduced heart rate variability on risk for cardiac events: The Framingham Heart Study. *Circulation, 94,* 2850-2855.

Wade, J. F. (1990). *The effects of the Callahan phobia treatment technique on self-concepts.* Unpublished doctoral dissertation, California School of Professional Psychology, San Diego, CA.

APPENDIX

Extended Trauma Protocol

Step 1. **Rate the Upset** on a One to Ten Scale as you think of situation (1 = no upset, 10 = worst)

Step 2. **Tap each point 10 times using fingertips: Side of hand, under nose, beginning of eyebrow, under eye, under arm, under collarbone, little finger, under collarbone, index finger, and under collarbone.**
   Do the 9 Gamut series. While continuously tapping the gamut spot:
   1. Close eyes
   2. Open eyes
   3. With your eyes look down and left
   4. With your eyes look down and right

5. Whirl your eyes in a complete circle in one direction
6. Whirl your eyes in a complete circle in the other direction
7. Hum a couple bars of any tune
8. Count to five
9. Hum again.

Repeat tapping each point 10 times using fingertips: Side of hand, under nose, beginning of eyebrow, under eye, under arm, under collarbone, little finger, index finger, and under collarbone.

Step 3. **Rate the upset:**
If upset is *two or less* on the ten point scale–**go to step 4.**
If upset is *not changed or has changed but has not dropped to two points* on the ten point scale–**repeat steps 2 and 3**. Stop if the upset is not dropping after repeating this several times.

Step 4. **Do the floor to ceiling eye roll.** While continuously tapping the gamut spot and holding your head level, rotate your eyes on a vertical line from the floor to the ceiling over 6-7 seconds.

TFT Algorithm Treatment Points
Side of hand (below the little finger)
Beginning of eyebrow (where the eyebrow begins above the bridge of the nose)
Under arm (about 4" down from the arm pit; at the bra line for women)
Under eye (in line with the pupil, just below the rim of the eye socket bone)
Collarbone (1" down from the V of the neck and 1" over, either left or right)
Index finger (beside the nail, on the thumb side)
Little finger (beside the nail on the thumb side)
Gamut spot (between the knuckles of the little and ring fingers, and about 1/2" toward the wrist)

Emotional Freedom Techniques: A Safe Treatment Intervention for Many Trauma Based Issues

Garry A. Flint
Willem Lammers
Deborah G. Mitnick

SUMMARY. Callahan (1985) developed a procedure of tapping on acupressure points for treating mental problems. Craig and Fowlie (1995) modified Callahan's procedure to a simplified version called Emotional Freedom Techniques (EFT). EFT is easy to teach and is effective with symptoms of PTSD. This article presents EFT as an adjunct to the Critical Incident Stress Reduction debriefing procedures. The use of EFT in debriefings results in shorter and more thorough sessions. It often reduces the emotional pain of the debriefing. This paper provides complete instructions and safeguards for using EFT when debriefing in disaster situations and with other applications. Included are references for further reading and training. *[Article copies available for a fee from The Haworth Document Delivery Service: 1-800-HAWORTH. E-mail address: <docdelivery@haworthpress.com> Website: <http://www.HaworthPress.com> © 2006 by The Haworth Press, Inc. All rights reserved.]*

Address correspondence to Garry A. Flint, #5-2906 32nd Street, Vernon, BC, V1T 5M1, Canada.

[Haworth co-indexing entry note]: "Emotional Freedom Techniques: A Safe Treatment Intervention for Many Trauma Based Issues." Flint, Garry A., Willem Lammers, and Deborah G. Mitnick. Co-published simultaneously in *Journal of Aggression, Maltreatment & Trauma* (The Haworth Maltreatment & Trauma Press, an imprint of The Haworth Press, Inc.) Vol. 12, No. 1/2, 2006, pp. 125-150; and: *Trauma Treatment Techniques: Innovative Trends* (ed: Jacqueline Garrick, and Mary Beth Williams) The Haworth Maltreatment & Trauma Press, an imprint of The Haworth Press, Inc., 2006, pp. 125-150. Single or multiple copies of this article are available for a fee from The Haworth Document Delivery Service [1-800-HAWORTH, 9:00 a.m. - 5:00 p.m. (EST). E-mail address: docdelivery@haworthpress.com].

Available online at http://www.haworthpress.com/web/JAMT
doi:10.1300/J146v12n01_07

KEYWORDS. Critical incident stress reduction, Emotional Freedom Technique, tapping, trauma, acupressure, PTSD, disaster, grief

Craig and Fowlie (1995) developed a technique for neutralizing traumatic memories called Emotional Freedom Techniques (EFT). In this treatment intervention, the patient taps on acupuncture points to neutralize the emotions associated with a traumatic experiences or beliefs. Because EFT is a very safe and simple method to learn and use, it was initially taught as a personal performance technique. In clinical practice, EFT has been shown to be effective for the treatment of many trauma-based issues. It is a useful intervention for mental health professionals and paraprofessionals to use, as well as for sharing among friends and family. This article is intended to teach the method at a practical level, thereby enabling the reader to experiment with it. In addition, the reader will be instructed in ways to integrate the EFT method with Critical Incident Stress Debriefing (CISD; Mitchell & Everly, 1996). The use of EFT often allows debriefings to be much shorter and thorough and often reduces the emotional pain of the debriefing.

OVERVIEW

Background and History

EFT is a modification of Callahan's (1985) Thought Field Therapy (TFT). Callahan studied Applied Kinesiology and extended the work of Goodheart (1964-78) and Diamond (1985) to mental health issues. Callahan discovered that muscle-testing points on each of the twelve major acupuncture meridians while the patient was thinking about a specific issue allows one to identify the sequence of acupressure points associated with that issue. His work led to the development of standardized sequences of acupressure points to use with issues typically seen in his students and clients. Roger Craig, one of Callahan's students, however, discovered that the sequences used were usually not important and that results similar to Callahan's could be obtained simply by tapping on all twelve acupressure points (Craig, 2000a). This finding greatly simplified the procedure for application and teaching.

There are many theories explaining the treatment process in EFT. It seems relatively clear that it is a learning process because change occurs; however, the mechanism of the active ingredients of change, like EMDR, are not yet known. Energy psychologists believe that the change process has to do with altering body energies that are represented in the meridians, while Flint (1994) believes that change is caused by a learning process triggered by stimulation. In either case, the EFT intervention works extremely well.

Efficacy Research

Presently, research on the efficacy of TFT and EFT remains sparse. Due to lack of quality research demonstrating the effectiveness of these treatment methods, both TFT and EFT are still considered to be experimental interventions. However, preliminary studies have offered promising results. Carbonell and Figley (1999), for example, carried out a three-year research project in which they tried to find out the active ingredients of therapeutic change among four therapies, including TFT. Results of this study suggested that TFT was as effective, if not more so, than the other more proved therapies examined. Figley (1995) stated that TFT was extraordinarily powerful, easily taught, and can produce fast and long lasting results, and did no harm. They also concluded that it was a successful treatment method in most of the trauma cases treated regardless of the exact tapping sequence used by the practitioner. In addition, Craig (2000a) believes there is no difference between the effectiveness of EFT and TFT.

Callahan and Callahan (2000, p. 50) cite two studies, each with 68 subjects, that involved treating phobias and anxieties over the telephone therapy while on radio talk shows. Callahan did the first unpublished study in 1986 for which he used a standard tapping algorithm for treatment. Leonoff (1995, p. 1), then, repeated Callahan's study in a different way. He used Voice Technology (VT) to determine over the telephone the exact treatment sequence for the caller's issue. The results of Leonoff's study published with Callahan's results were almost identical with Callahan's original study (Callahan & Callahan, 2000, p. 50). The average decrease in experienced distress for treated participants was 74% or better, and the average amount of time needed to achieve the results was less than 6.04 minutes, which indicates that TFT causes changes very quickly. TFT and EFT practitioners often find similar rapid results in their clinical practices.

Recently, Andrade and Feinstein (2002, p. 2) published preliminary results of in-house studies of the tapping therapies, TFT and EFT, based on 29,000 patients. Overall, they found better than 70% effectiveness with the tapping treatment. An additional study compared tapping treatment versus Cognitive Behavior Therapy with medication (CBT/M; Andrade & Feinstein, 2002, p. 3). The study extended over a five-and-one-half year period ($N = 5000$), and looked at anxiety disorders, including diagnoses of panic, agoraphobia, social phobias, specific phobias, obsessive compulsive disorders, generalized anxiety disorders, PTSD, and acute stress disorders; and somatoform disorders, eating disorders, ADHD, and addiction disorders. The patients, selected from 11 clinics in Uruguay and Argentina, were randomly assigned to each group. The data collected on these patients were intake history, record of the procedures used, clinical responses and double-blind follow-up interviews by telephone or in person at one, three, six, and twelve months. Positive responses to treatment "ranging from complete relief to partial relief to short relief with relapses" were found in 63% of the CBT/M group and 90% of the tapping group. Further, 52% of the CBT/M group and 76% of the tapping group found complete relief from symptoms.

Andrade and Feinstein (2002, p. 4) cite another study that compared CBT/M to a tapping/dissociation treatment in assessing the number of treatment sessions to completion ($N = 200$). In the latter group, tapping and VK dissociation techniques were used as needed. VK dissociation involves the patient viewing the trauma as a movie while manipulating sensory qualities of the movie by imagining a tactile, color, or auditory distortion. The results showed that it took an average of 15 sessions for the CBT/M group and an average of 3 sessions for the tapping/dissociation group. The results of these studies suggest the tapping treatment is safe, effective, and efficient.

EFT Is a Practical Treatment Method

EFT is a treatment method that is easy to learn (Craig & Fowlie, 1995). This treatment is effective with most anxiety or trauma based issues, has remarkable effect with pain by treating remembered pain that contributes to chronic pain, is extremely safe, easy to teach, is a natural self-help treatment intervention (Callahan & Callahan, 2000; Durlacher, 1994; Flint, 2001), and can be taught to and used voluntarily by children. The effects of EFT treatment are usually immediately experienced and are long lasting.

The information given in this article will be sufficient to treat many trauma-based issues. More extensive instruction is available from a manual and videotape course produced by Craig and Fowlie (1995) as well as the book entitled *Emotional Freedom* (Flint, 2001), which presents the content of Craig and Foulie's (1995) videotape course. Craig's (2000b) Web site has case histories of many mental and physical issues.

Treatment with EFT is usually very effective and reliable (Craig & Fowlie, 1995, p. 114). The worst that can happen seems to be that the treatment method does not work. Very few clients report getting upset when tapping acupuncture points (Craig & Fowlie, 1995, p. 39). In such cases when upsets occur, the meridian acupressure points can be stimulated through touching or breathing to reduce the intensity of the emotional pain (Diepold, 2000). With clients who have complex trauma, psychosis, and Dissociative Identity Disorder, EFT should be not be used as a stand-alone treatment technique and cannot replace long-term psychotherapy. In this case, it can be an additional tool once the therapeutic relationship has been firmly established. The authors recommend that only professional therapists treat persons in acute crisis, persons who are currently in therapy, or those who have a history of hospitalizations.

Skill Level Required

Non-clinicians can be taught to use EFT. Therapists routinely teach their clients to use EFT and TFT on themselves at home. These clients often report that they were able to teach relatives to effectively use and benefit from this technique. In all cases, common sense precautions should be used. If the person using EFT experiences intense fear or negative emotions while being treated by a layperson, the method should be terminated and the client should be advised to find a professional therapist.

EFT may also be a useful adjunct to CISD, as mental health workers, nurses, clergy, and others who conduct CISD sessions can use it. CISD involves cognitive debriefings in which survivors are able to share and verbalize their experiences, with the support of fellow survivors, and process the traumatic events in a healthy way (Mitchell & Everly, 1996). Used as a tool for reducing traumatic stress, therefore, EFT may be a particularly useful after initial crisis counseling.

EFT, however, cannot replace psychotherapy for the treatment of severe trauma. Therefore, when persons are suffering from PTSD or are in crisis, the mental health worker will still need to develop rapport with the client, take a brief history, assess suicidal risk, and rule out dissociative processes. These persons should be carefully evaluated to determine whether a referral to a professional psychotherapist is appropriate.

INSTRUCTIONS FOR USING THE EFT METHOD

Basic Recipe for Using EFT

There are basically two steps to learning and using EFT. First, one must learn to identify the issues and aspects with which to work. Second, one must learn the EFT treatment method itself. The goal of the first step is to identify the important aspects of each issue presented by the client, to describe them in a sentence, and to then generate a reminder phrase. The goal of the reminder phrase is to help the client keep focused on the emotional content of the issue during the treatment. The second step (i.e., to learn the treatment method) involves tapping on acupressure points. There are two methods. The first is a sequence that requires tapping on 12 acupressure points. The second, the 9-Gamut, requires tapping on the back of the hand and doing eye movements and vocalizing. This will be described in detail later. The EFT method can be used to treat the important aspects of any issue.

When learning the EFT tapping intervention, the mental health worker must follow the treatment instructions very carefully. The authors recommend memorizing the basic steps of EFT, which are as follows: (a) Forming the positive affirmation joined with a reminder phrase, or a phrase that keeps the issue in your thoughts; (b) Measuring the emotional intensity of the issue or aspect on a scale ranging from 0 to 10; (c) Applying the affirmation or modified affirmation; (d) Tapping on acupressure points described later as the sequence, the 9-Gamut treatment, and then repeating the sequence; (e) Troubleshooting when the healing process has stopped; and (f) Doing steps b through e (i.e., a treatment cycle) until the emotional level of the issue or aspect is reduced to a scale of zero (Flint, 2001, p. 33). Some steps in this "basic recipe" can occasionally be omitted without losing effectiveness (Flint, 2001, p. 36). However, it is recommended that the complete EFT method be used to insure maximum effectiveness both when learning it and when using it in situations where contact with the clients may be time limited.

Identifying Aspects of the Issues for Treatment

Clients will have issues with multiple aspects that have to be treated (Flint, 2001, p. 15). For this reason, it is always useful to ask if there are any other beliefs or experiences that are related to the issues identified by the client. The mental health worker should have the client write down all aspects of the issue chosen for treatment as descriptive sentences and include key words, for example, "I feel empty with all my losses." It is important to describe each aspect of the issue as specifically as possible.

Furthermore, when obtaining descriptive sentences of aspects, the mental health professional should focus on specific visual or auditory perceptions ("my cat's eyes," or "the breathing of the victim next to me,") or use a description of the emotion in its context ("My fear, when I saw the truck driving into the train."). In addition, the emotions should be described as adjectives, rather than as nouns (e.g., not "emptiness" but "empty"; not "anger" but "angry"). Emotions are active processes. The authors believe that when nouns are used to describe emotions, they seem to consolidate and become less accessible. Using an adjective, a process word, suggests and maintains active emotions, which allows for rapid treatment.

The descriptive sentence will then be used to elicit the emotion associated with the related aspect of the issue being treated. Through the use of such descriptive sentences, the mental health worker is able to get a measure of the pretreatment intensity of the painful emotion elicited by the individual aspects of the issue. Each individual aspect or component of a larger issue may include memories that are visual, auditory, tactile, or olfactory in nature. They may also include beliefs and emotions associated with the loss of tangible items.

Treating the individual aspects of a trauma with EFT often leads to rapid positive change (Craig & Fowlie, 1995, p. 70). When there is no change in one's thinking or emotional reactivity toward some aspect of the trauma, the aspect can become a new issue to be treated because of its complexity. In such cases, the new issue becomes independent of the original trauma issue from which it came and needs to be treated separately. The new issue may be found to have multiple aspects to treat.

Appropriate Issues for Treatment

In the initial stage of learning the method, EFT can be used on oneself, family, and friends. Initially, the mental health worker can try it on simple phobias, such as a fear of public speaking or spiders. Avoid phobias based upon severe trauma, such as a phobia caused by a severe accident or by an animal attack. For some people, thinking about these phobias generates emotions that may be difficult for a beginner to handle or may be beyond their initial skill level. As confidence builds, EFT can be used on other less painful issues or aspects. When confidence is strong, the mental health worker can use EFT on more difficult issues and aspects.

In disaster situations, for example, the mental health provider should try to keep the treatment focused on the specific trauma of the disaster rather than on the general emotions elicited by the event. This is done to avoid triggering old traumas associated with those emotions. The focus of treatment can be better controlled if the disaster is treated as a movie and the treatment focuses only on the emotions and memories associated with each traumatic frame of that movie. The frames of the movie become different aspects of the disaster that can be safely treated separately (Flint, 2001, p. 15). For example, the emotion "terror" could be connected not only to the disaster being discussed, but also to other events from the client's past. Therefore, focusing on the emotion of "terror," rather than on the specifics of the disaster situation, may leave the client vulnerable to being traumatized by memories associated with any past event that was also experienced as terrifying. Therefore, to keep the client focused on the presenting trauma, the client's reminder phrase should be specific to the current trauma (e.g., "terror of the forest fire"). Also, by focusing on the specific "frames" depicting the event (e.g., "the exploding tree") all of the emotions connected to this frame can be neutralized during the EFT process. The goal of treatment is to allow the client to be able to look neutrally at the mental pictures (frames) depicting the disaster situation (e.g., the exploding tree).

The following vignette is a clinical example of the application of this strategy. A railroad engineer witnessed another man's suicide. The man was sitting between the rails and looked directly into the eyes of the engineer as the train ran over him. EFT treatment focused on the client's view of the man's eyes prior to the crash and body parts after the crash. After using EFT, the engineer was able to remember the incident calmly, saying: "It was his choice, I couldn't help it."

The Reminder Phase

Once the aspects of a chosen issue are identified, a reminder phrase is designed to keep the trauma memory active so that tapping treatment can effectively change the memory. When you are not thinking about the issue, the trauma memory is not active. The memory of the issue has to be active for the treatment process to work. Saying the reminder phrase keeps the memory of the trauma issue active. Expanding on the above forest fire example, the specific aspects associated with this trauma can be organized into those depicted in Table 1.

TABLE 1. Traumatic Aspects Associated with Forest Fire Example

Issue	Aspect	Reminder Phrase for
Aspect		
The forest fire exploding tree	I have flashbacks to the fire.	That
	I feel empty with all my losses.	Empty
	I feel grief over the loss of my cat.	My cat grief
	I can still smell the situation.	That smell
	I feel devastated by losing my home.	This loss

Obtaining a Measure of Emotional Intensity

Obtaining a measure of emotional intensity is the first step in EFT treatment. The mental health worker has the client measure the intensity of his or her distress over the chosen issue on the Subjective Units of Distress (SUD) scale. This self-report measure was used in Eye Movement Desensitization and Reprocessing (EMDR; Shapiro, 1995, p. 70). A SUD level of 0 indicates no emotional distress, while a SUD level at 10 is very intense emotional distress. Having clients periodically rate their level of distress on the 11-point SUD scale allows the mental health worker to detect changes in the client's or group's subjective experience of trauma symptoms as treatment progresses.

When working with an individual, the mental health worker initially asks the client to estimate the SUD that best describes the intensity of his or her emotion after reciting the descriptive statement created for each aspect of the issue being treated. Guessing is acceptable when the client is unable to estimate the level of distress that the statement will elicit, since it is a subjective measure and a guess is as good as anything. These estimations or guesses provide a baseline level of emotional distress for that issue. Then, after each treatment cycle, the SUD level is reassessed to monitor the effects of the treatment. Assessing emotional intensity is an important part of EFT treatment because a comparison of the client's SUD scores is used to determine whether to stop the treatment, to do another treatment cycle, or to troubleshoot by using corrections to remove the barrier blocking the effectiveness of the treatment when no change in the level of distress is detected.

When conducting CISD with groups, the debriefer introduces the concept of the SUD measure at the beginning of the group CISD process. The debriefer has the participants monitor their own SUD levels during the formal CISD process by asking for a show of hands for different intervals of SUD levels (e.g., 9 to 10, 7 to 8, etc.). The debriefer keeps a tally of the number of group members that endorse each interval. This process is repeated periodically throughout the debriefing. The changing tally shows the group members the effectiveness of the CISD process and indicates those members who are still having problems. This protocol may also set the stage for introducing EFT as another method to further lower the SUD levels.

It is important to be flexible and adjust your treatment intervention to the level of emotions and the needs of the group. When appropriate, you can introduce the SUD measure to track change. This stimulates interest and curiosity about the outcome of the treatment process. By learning to assess and record the SUD level for the aspect being addressed after each treatment cycle, the focus of treatment can be returned to later in the process if it changes before the aspect is fully healed (i.e., a SUD rating of 0 is obtained). In this way, the mental health worker can honor the client's experience and tailor the treatment to the needs of the client or group in order to provide thorough treatment.

THE TREATMENT METHOD

Affirmation

An affirmation is a self-empowering statement that precedes one's stated acceptance of the emotions associated with the issue or aspect. The statement strengthens the client's self-acceptance and is used to correct most barriers for healing (Flint, 2001, p. 20). When reciting the chosen affirmation, the client should press hard enough to find a sore spot on his/her chest, about 3 inches down and 3 inches over from the notch in the neck (see Figure 1). The sore spot is then rubbed continu-

FIGURE 1. Locating a Sore Spot

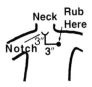

ously while the client repeats the phrase: "I accept myself even though I have this [*insert reminder phrase*]" three times. Other affirmations that can be used are as follows: (a) "I'm OK even if [*insert reminder phrase*]"; (b) "I deeply and profoundly accept myself even if [*insert reminder phrase*]"; or (c) "I love and accept myself even if [*insert reminder phrase*]" (Flint, 2001, p. 20). The reminder phrase is also said aloud when tapping on the acupressure points.

Modified Affirmation

The modified affirmation is used after the first treatment and when the SUD level stops reducing in intensity (Flint, 2001, p. 22). In this case, the affirmation is modified slightly by including words that emphasize the continuing intensity of an issue. When the SUD level stops going down, a barrier is believed to be stopping the healing process. When this happens, the client should do the entire treatment again, including the modified affirmation. The modified affirmation is also recited three times while rubbing on the sore spot on the chest, and includes statements such as: "I accept myself even though I **still** have some of this **remaining** [*reminder phrase*]." The words in bold are the important words to include and emphasize in the modified affirmation. Again, the client says the "**remaining** [*reminder phrase*]" aloud when tapping on the acupressure points.

The Acupressure Point Sequence

The acupressure point sequence consists of tapping five to seven times on each of twelve acupressure meridian points (Flint, 2001, p. 25). The tapping should be firm enough to hear the tap, but not firm enough to hurt. The client taps with the index and middle finger of each hand and simultaneously repeats a reminder phrase aloud to remind one of the content or emotion associated with the issue or aspect of the issue being treated. The 9-gamut sequence, described later, is done after the acupressure point sequence. This sequence is also tapped. Once it is completed, the acupressure point sequence is tapped again.

The twelve acupressure meridian points of the acupressure point sequence are as follows:

1. *Eyebrow*–Guide the client to locate both spots at the beginning of the eyebrow near the bridge of the nose (see Figure 2). Use both

hands to tap on both sides. Be sure the tapping spots are near the bridge of the nose. Have the client tap 5 to 7 times on those spots.

2. *Outer Eye*–Have the client locate the spot on the bone next to the outside corner of the eye (see Figure 3). Make sure the client taps on the spot adjacent to the corner of the eye. Tap 5 to 7 times on those spots on the bone with both hands.

3. *Under the Eye*–Locate the spot on the bone under the eye, directly below the pupil (see Figure 4). Guide the client to locate the right spots. Tap on those spots 5 to 7 times using both hands.

4. *Under the Nose*–Have the client find the spot under the nose (see Figure 5) and tap on it with the index and middle fingers using only one hand.

5. *Under the Lip*–Have the client find the spot under the lower lip on the indent area of the chin (see Figure 5) and tap. Again, use one hand.

6. *Collarbone*–This point may be a little more difficult to find. Have the client locate the notch at the top of the chest bone, at the base of the throat (see Figure 6). Have her put their fingers there and move them down 1 inch and, then, over 1 inch on the right and left sides of her chest. Be sure her fingers are only 2 inches apart. These are the collarbone spots. They are located on a depression under the joint of each collarbone. Have her tap on these spots with both hands.

7. *Under the Arm*–Now the client will tap on a spot 4 inches under the underarms (see Figure 7). For a woman, this spot is found on the bra material over the ribs. For a man, this spot is level with the nipple. They can cross their arms over the body to tap with their fingers or raise their arms and tap with their thumbs. Tap 5 to 7 times.

   Next, the client will be asked to tap on four fingers and on the edge of her left hand, one spot at a time. Instruct the client to tap 5 to 7 times on each spot. Figure 8 depicts the index finger of the left hand facing down so the client can clearly identify the location of the base of the fingernail. The client will be tapping on her fingers next to the base of the fingernail on the inside of each finger on the spot closest to her body. Have her carefully look at the pictures of the left-hand fingers, palm facing down, and follow the instructions. Incidentally, one can tap with either hand.

8. *Thumb*–Have her find the spot on the inside of the thumb closest to the body (see Figure 9). Then have her tap on the skin next to the base of the thumbnail.

9. *Index Finger*–Have her find the spot on the inside of the index finger. The spot is on the skin next to the base of the fingernail on the same side of the thumb (see Figure 10). Have her tap.
10. *Middle Finger*–Have her find the spot on the inside of the middle finger on the skin next to the base of the fingernail (see Figure 11). Have her tap. After tapping, skip the ring finger and go to the little finger.
11. *Little Finger*–Have her find the spot on the inside of the little finger on the skin next to the base of the fingernail (see Figure 12). Again, have her tap.
12. *Karate Chop*–Help her locate the spot on center of the soft skin on the outside edge of her left hand between the knuckle of the little finger and the knuckle of the wrist (see Figure 13). Have her tap this spot 5 to 7 times.

FIGURE 2. The Eyebrow

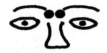

FIGURE 3. The Outer Eye

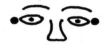

FIGURE 4. Under the Eye

FIGURE 5. Under the Nose and Lip

FIGURE 6. The Collarbone

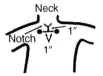

FIGURE 7. Under the Arm

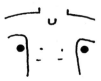

FIGURE 8. Locating the Base of the Fingernail

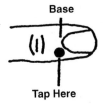

FIGURE 9. The Thumb

FIGURE 10. The Index Finger

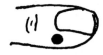

FIGURE 11. The Middle Finger

The 9-Gamut Tapping Sequence

The 9-Gamut (Flint, 2001, p. 30) involves tapping rapidly on the back of the hand while following nine instructions (below). It takes some practice because the activity is like patting your head and rubbing your stomach at the same time. First, have the client find the spot on the back of either hand that is half an inch back from the knuckles of both the ring finger and little finger (see Figure 14) and tap rapidly on that spot while following the instructions described below.

While the client taps the back of the hand rapidly, have the client hold his or her head upright and do the following nine steps (Figures 15-23).

The 9-Gamut should be practiced until it can be done easily. To assist the client in learning EFT, the help sheet can be obtained online from http://www.emotional-freedom.com/files/helpsheet.pdf or http://www.emotional-freedom.com/helpsheet.htm.

FIGURE 12. The Little Finger

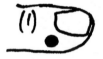

FIGURE 13. The Karate Chop

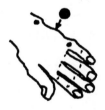

FIGURE 14. Locating the Spot on the Back of the Hand

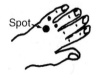

FIGURE 15. Close Eyes

FIGURE 16. Open Eyes

FIGURE 17. Looking Down to the Left

FIGURE 18. Looking Down to the Right

FIGURE 19. Circle the Eyes One Way

FIGURE 20. Circle the Eyes the Other Way

FIGURE 21. Humming Out Loud

FIGURE 22. Counting from 1 to 5

Say: "1, 2, 3, 4, 5"

FIGURE 23. Humming Out Loud Again

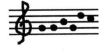

A SUMMARY OF THE WHOLE INTERVENTION

To use the EFT treatment intervention with groups or individuals, the recipient(s) must be both prepared for the method and guided through the treatment process. To prepare one for EFT, the mental health worker helps the client to choose an issue, identify the important aspects of that issue, and develop reminder phrases for each of the aspects identified. In addition, preparation for this treatment method involves familiarizing one with the acupressure point sequence and 9-Gamut sequence that will be used during the course of the treatment process. In the preparation phase, the mental health worker helps the recipient(s) to do the following: (a) Identify the most bothersome target issue; (b) Inquire about other aspects of the issue that may be relevant; (c) List the aspects from least intense to the most intense; and (d) Obtain reminder phrases that are clearly related to the issues and aspects.

EFT treatment requires the client to tap on the acupressure points. It involves having the client cycle the EFT process for each aspect of the issue until the SUD level reported for each is reduced to 0 or close to 0. When using EFT with individuals or groups, the mental health provider must guide the recipient(s) through a series of steps, listed in Table 2.

TROUBLESHOOTING BARRIERS TO HEALING

If the SUD level stops decreasing, the client has hit a barrier to progress. Several examples of barriers are traumatic aspects, oppositional beliefs, a physiological condition that stops learning, dehydration, or the presence of an odor in the environment. All of these will stop the treatment process. There are several ways to remove a barrier blocking the treatment process (Flint, 2001, p. 38). To troubleshoot, the mental health worker instructs the client to try each of a number of commonly used corrections, in the order presented below, until they find the one that removes the barrier. Removal of the barrier is indicated by a decrease in the SUD level. The six most frequently used corrections to treatment barriers in EFT, which have been listed according to their likelihood of being utilized in disaster applications, are listed below (see Flint, 2001, p. 38, for the entire list).

> 1. *Modified Affirmation.* If the modified affirmation was not said, have the client do the method again and include the modified affirmation. The affirmation is the first part of the method and is specifi-

cally used to correct barriers that frequently inhibit progress. Sometimes, it may be necessary to use the modified affirmation with every application of the treatment cycle. In some cases, the emotional intensity measure will go down only one SUD level at a time.

2. *Review the Issue.* If the issue being focused on has a number of aspects, attempting to obtain therapeutic gains by focusing on only one aspect of the issue may not work. Therefore, other aspects related to the issue may need to be addressed individually. Often the client may need to get more specific when describing an issue in order to assure that all of the important aspects are addressed. For example, with the issue "survived the forest fire," the aspects may be "fear of death," "fear of suffocating," "death of my cat," etc. Each of these aspects may contribute to the client's distress over the forest fire.

3. *A Brain Condition.* A form of brain disorganization is allegedly caused by neurological disorganization in the brain that prevents the change process (Durlacher, 1995, p. 48). As strange as it seems, by placing the back of the hand on the chest (see Figure 24) and then by tapping on the palm five times, this barrier is corrected (Flint, 2001, p. 40). Sometimes, if change is very slow, doing this correction before the modified affirmation causes more rapid change.

4. *Drink Water.* Sometimes our electrolyte balance is poor. Have the client drink eight ounces of water and try the method again.

5. *Change Location.* Environmental factors, such as the smell of perfume or industrial solvents, may cause brain disorganization and stop the treatment process (Flint, 2001, p. 41). Having the client move to another location, such as the kitchen, the bathroom, outside, or elsewhere to try the method moves the client away from the chemical causing the barrier. If trying the method in another place works, then some chemical or property of the environment may have been causing the barrier. Taking a shower without soap may also correct this kind of barrier at times (Craig & Fowlie, 1995, p. 129).

6. *Patience and Persistence.* Some issues require the client to keep repeating the EFT treatment cycle several times per day. Having patience and being persistent by continuing the treatment on a routine basis over days may be necessary for success, particularly with recurring symptoms. Patience and persistence are required to complete the troubleshooting process, as well.

TABLE 2. Sequence of Steps of EFT

1. Unless contraindicated, have the client select the most bothersome issue or aspect.

2. Assess the starting SUD level of the emotions associated with the aspect.

3. While the client is rubbing the sore spot on her chest, she says the affirmation out loud 3 times.

4. The client then does the sequence. Have her tap on each acupressure point 5-7 times, repeating the reminder phrase out loud for each acupressure point.

5. The client is instructed to think of the reminder phrase and do the entire 9-Gamut treatment.

6. Then have the client repeat the sequence by tapping on each acupressure point 5-7 times, repeating the reminder phrase out loud for each point.

7. Reassess the SUD level of the emotions attached to the aspect.

8. If the SUD level drops more than 2 points, have the client repeat the treatment cycle. If the SUD level stops going down, have the client use a modified affirmation as described above, and repeat the whole EFT treatment cycle 1 to 7. If it still does not decrease, the mental health worker will troubleshoot with the client.

FIGURE 24. Location of Tapping Correction for a Brain Condition

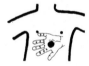

USING EFT IN A DISASTER SITUATION

Immediately after a traumatic event, most survivors need additional emotional and cognitive resources to manage their experience. The contribution a mental health worker offers is a secure relationship with clients. This relationship allows the clients both to reorient themselves in the face of the events and deal with practical issues such as accessing money, telephoning relatives, and dealing with household pets. The survivors' needs should direct the nature of the support and interventions offered during this time. Such logistical and emotional support can help clients regain the resources needed to cope with a traumatic experience.

When survivors have reached a more or less stable state, they can be asked individually or in a group to tell their stories. At this point, the mental health worker can get information about the symptoms related to re-experiencing, avoidance, and heightened arousal that may emerge following a trauma. Examples of this information might be a verbal statement, a change in color, tearing, or a change in the vocal quality, like a shaky voice or a voice driven by painful emotion. Any of these examples would indicate that person was still distressed by the trauma and needed further attention. Groups and individuals are handled somewhat differently.

Working with Groups

When the expression of painful emotions has subsided and the attendees are less disorganized, a CISD group meeting can be held. CISD is not considered to be therapy, but is a part of the Critical Incident Stress Management process. It is a method used to help people process normal reactions to abnormal events. However, not all survivors should be put in the same group; it is important that those within a group have had a similar experience of the trauma. For example, those who witnessed a murder, those who heard the shots and saw the dead body or bodies, and those who were somewhere else in the building should be placed in separate CISD groups to avoid further traumatizing survivors with explicit details of the event that they did not experience personally. Similarly, the mental health worker should identify early in the process any clients who would rather be seen privately or who would benefit from being treated separately.

The CISD cognitive debriefing process encourages each member to express what he or she saw, heard, felt, smelled, tasted, thought, and did. For many clients, symptoms will be relieved in the course of the debriefing process. Some, however, will need further therapeutic support (e.g., individual psychotherapy or participation in an ongoing support group) to process the event. Social support facilitates processing, while therapist intrusion, irritability, and helplessness may inhibit it (Freedman & Shalev, 2000, p. 250). Several pretrauma variables have been shown to predict PTSD, such as child abuse, physical abuse, intelligence, and socioeconomic status (Freedman & Shalev, 2000, p. 250).

Therefore, while the goal of CISD is to stay focused on the presenting trauma, sometimes the processing of earlier material is unavoidable.

Using SUD measures to keep track of survivors' emotional distress during the debriefing progress adds to the CISD process. In addition, it is by the use of SUD levels that the mental health worker can introduce EFT as an adjunct to the CISD or individual debriefing process. The SUD measure should be defined early in the session and, using the approach described above, SUD ratings for various aspects of the trauma should be obtained both early in the session and a number of times throughout the CISD process. In addition, it is important for the mental health worker to be aware of the presenting problems that were precipitated by the traumatic event and to address specific incidents or emotions in order to track change and recognize when the symptom's intensity has been reduced or resolved. If, during the CISD process, survivors have had the opportunity to build a working relationship with the mental health worker and share their experiences, the movement between SUD levels will usually indicate a reduction in the stress connected to the event. A visible sign of symptom reduction (i.e., reduction in the SUD ratings) not only generates and maintains the group's interest in the process, but also provides the mental health worker with an opening to reveal the option to use EFT.

If the mental health worker has established solid rapport with the group, s/he can effectively introduce EFT to survivors at the end of the formal CISD as a method for further symptom reduction. The group should be asked if any of its members have experience with EFT and, if applicable, whether their experience was positive. At this stage (e.g., the second or third meeting in the "Utrecht" model [Kleber & Brom, 1992, p. 94]), EFT can be introduced as an additional technique to help the client overcome the trauma by further reducing the SUD level associated with various aspects of it, without the in-depth re-experiencing of the event. Before using EFT, the clients must feel safe within the context of the relationship with the practitioner and the group. By the end of the process, the group may be ready to accept EFT as a gentle method to lower any remaining emotional intensity levels. If so, practitioners should specifically ask what symptom is still intense and focus their use of the EFT treatment to the identified area of concern.

Working with Individuals

When working with individual trauma survivors, distress about the various aspects of the traumatic event should first be measured in terms of SUD levels. Once rapport has been established, EFT can be introduced as a process to reduce emotional pain or as a means of lowering their ratings on the SUD scale. The mental health worker should listen for painful experiences, memories, pictures, or sounds associated with the traumatic event. Determine whether or not the client has negative or maladaptive beliefs, flashbacks, or auditory, visual, or olfactory intrusions. These internal events are caused by trauma and will need treatment. With each issue, look for other beliefs or associated aspects that are related to the issue. The aspect that is most bothersome to the client should be selected for EFT treatment. Once resolved, the remaining aspects can be systematically treated in order of the level of distress they are causing.

When the experience unfolds in a sequence of traumas, in some cases it may be appropriate to heal from the most recent trauma in the sequence and then work backwards to the first trauma of the sequence. This is done for several reasons. The most recent trauma is usually less threatening than the initial trauma. The initial trauma often has happened at a time when coping skills were not yet fully developed because of lack of life experience. If the treatment begins with the first trauma of the sequence, the later traumas may be triggered resulting in emotional flooding. Also, if the last traumatic experience is not the worst and is addressed first, the client can learn that the trauma of an event can be resolved.

After a number of rounds of EFT, the client will be ready to tell the "story" of the traumatic incident. If the client can tell the story from beginning to end without any distress, treatment can be considered complete. If, however, the client experiences any residual emotional distress as s/he reports the details, continuation of the EFT treatment is indicated for the aspects of the story that are causing the emotional experience.

In ongoing crisis situations, if acceptable to the client, EFT can be used to stabilize the client's flood of emotions, as well as to process aspects of the traumatic events. In situations where the threat of disaster is ongoing or pending, the use of EFT can help the client to think more rationally and protect themselves better. For example, EFT is effective with either individual or group treatment in situations or countries with ongoing violence (P. Cane, personal communication, April 16, 2002).

CASE STUDIES

Case 1

A therapist was asked to conduct a Critical Incident Stress Debriefing (CISD) for 35 members of an organization where an employee had died (Mitnick, 1998). The formal CISD session was 90-minutes long. During the session, the therapist continually assessed if EFT would be an appropriate intervention. After the therapist introduced herself, she set the ground rules for the session and described the seven-step CISD process. She also set the stage for the possibility of using EFT by telling the participants that, if they experienced any emotional distress, she could teach them a method that would provide quick relaxation and would most likely diminish the intensity of their distress. The SUD scale was explained and initial scores were obtained after the explanation. Group distribution of SUD scores indicated a few participants at 8-9, most at 5-6, and a few at 3-4. SUD level reassessment was done after each of the seven steps in the CISD process and levels of intensity diminished for most participants at each step. This process of self-evaluation kept participants in close touch with their emotions, clearly revealed their progress, and reminded them of their options for further support. Most participants in the formal CISD had significantly lower scores (SUDS ranging from 3 to 0) by the end of that session.

Six participants asked for additional individual EFT assistance and found rapid relief by using this method. Following the CISD session, the six participants who requested EFT formed a small group. These participants were still feeling intense about the death during the formal CISD, but after the tapping of EFT in the small group setting, they had significantly reduced SUDS to between 2 and 0. The EFT session was very brief and only one or two aspects were dealt with for each participant. Of course, everyone had a slightly different experience of the trauma since they all came from different life experiences, but as a group, their relationship with the deceased was the same. EFT was, for them, an appropriate intervention for more completely reducing and eliminating traumatic memories after a formal CISD session.

Case 2

The second author treated a client who was traumatized from an accident that occurred while working on a moving train. While the crew tried to connect a line of railway cars to a single stationary car at the end of the track, a coworker was riding on the last moving car. The client was receiving instructions from this coworker by means of a short wave radio when he suddenly heard, via the radio, the voice of his colleague exclaiming: "They got me!" The train had been moving too fast and the car on which his colleague was riding collided with the stationary car. His colleague was severely injured and lost his foot.

Six years later, the client still experienced intrusions of the voice of his coworker and still experienced significant guilt about his coworker's injury. Twenty minutes of CISD processing was spent on the accident. This reduced the SUD level for the intrusion of the memories of his coworker's voice from an 8 to 4. The CISD process also helped the client to build a working relationship by showing the client that the practitioner believed him and took him seriously. This made it relatively easy to introduce and use EFT. After processing the trauma with EFT, the client's SUD score dropped to zero after only a few treatments. Following treatment, the client's guilt was also considerably reduced and he could see that it was his colleague, not he, who had made the mistake.

Eight months after he received treatment during an EFT training for railway relief workers, the client wrote that he has asked himself repeatedly what he was so troubled about during those six years. He added that there are no symptoms connected to the event now, and he was able to tell the story without negative emotions or bodily symptoms. In his "mind's eye," it was as if the memory of the situation had dissolved.

RECOMMENDATIONS FOR FUTURE STUDY

The following research could be done to enhance the use of EFT in disaster situations. Though it is inappropriate to use disaster survivors directly as identified experimental subjects in a research project, practitioners can obtain helpful data by developing and gathering data on a Case Results Form. The Case Results Form would obtain feedback as to how the CISD and EFT processes were introduced, how the group accepted the interventions, how the issues and aspects were identified, and how successful the CISD and EFT interventions were. Access to such forms would also allow researchers to compile a list of problematic issues typically facing disaster survivors. This data would increase our understanding of how to use EFT in disaster settings and would be helpful in creating an EFT treatment protocol based on data for using of EFT in complex disaster situations. For additional information concerning the use of EFT, please see the resources provided in the Appendix.

Author Note

Sections of this book are from *Emotional Freedom* (Rev. ed.) by Garry A. Flint, 2001, Vernon, BC, Canada: NeoSolTerric Enterprises. Copyright 2001 by Garry A. Flint. Adapted with permission.

REFERENCES

Andrade, J., & Feinstein, D. (2002). Energy psychology: Theory, indications, evidence. In D. Feinstein (Ed.), *Energy psychology interactive: An integrated book and CD program for learning the fundamentals of energy psychology.* Available at: http://www.innersource.net/energy_psych/epi_research.htm.

Callahan, R. J. (1985). *Five minute phobia cure.* Wilmington, DE: Enterprise Publishers.

Callahan, R. J. & Callahan, J. (2000). *Stop the nightmares of trauma.* Indian Wells, CA: Author.

Carbonell, J. L. & Figley, C. (1999). Promising PTSD treatment approaches: A systematic clinical demonstration of promising PTSD Treatment Approaches. *TRAUMATOLOGYe, 5*(1), Article 4. Retrieved March 1, 2004, from http://www.fsu.edu/~trauma/promising. html.

Craig, G. (2000a). *The evolution of EFT to TFTtm: Part I to V.* Retrieved March 1, 2004, from http://209.221.150.70/articles/scien-i.htm.

Craig, G. (2000b). *EFT cases on varied issues from the EFT e-mail support list.* Retrieved March 1, 2004, from http://www.emofree.com/cases/critical.htm.

Craig, G. & Fowlie, A. (1995). *Emotional freedom techniques: The manual (with video and audio tapes).* Sea Ranch, CA: Author.

Diamond, J. (1985). *Life energy.* New York: Dodd, Mead and Co.

Diepold, J. H., Jr. (2000). Touch and breathe (TAB): An alternative treatment approach with meridian-based psychotherapies. *Electronic Journal of Traumatology, 6*(2) Article 4. Retrieved March 1, 2004, from http://www.fsu.edu/~trauma/v6i2a4.html.

Durlacher, J. V. (1994). *Freedom from fear forever.* Tempe, AZ: Author.

Figley, C. R. (1995). *Letter to colleagues.* Retrieved March 1, 2004, from http://www.trauma-pages.com/tft.htm.

Flint, G. A. (2001). *Emotional freedom: Techniques for dealing with emotional and physical distress* (Rev. ed.). Vernon, British Columbia: NeoSolTerric Enterprises.

Freedman, S., & Shalev, A.Y. (2000). Prospective studies of the recently traumatized. In A. Y. Shalev, R. Yehuda, & A. C. McFarlane (Eds.), *International handbook of human response to trauma* (pp. 249-261). Dordrecht, Netherlands: Kluwer.

Goodheart, G. J., Jr. (1964-1978). *Applied kinesiology: Workshop method manual* (Ed. 1-14). Privately. Detroit, MI.

Kleber, R. J., Brom, D., & DeFares, P. B. (1992). *Coping with trauma: Theory, prevention and therapy.* Amsterdam/Lisse: Swets and Zeitlinger.

Leonoff, G. (1995). Successful treatment of phobias and anxiety by telephone and radio: A replication of Callahan's 1987 study. *The Thought Field Therapy Newsletter, 1*(2).

Mitchell, J. T., & Everly, G. S. (1996). *Critical Incident Stress Debriefing: An operations manual.* Ellicott City, MD: Chevron.

Mitnick, D. (1998). *Critical incident stress debriefing.* Retrieved March 1, 2004, from http://www.emofree.com/cases/critical.htm.

Shapiro, F. (1995). *Eye movement desensitization and reprocessing: Basic principles, protocols, and procedures.* New York: Guilford.

APPENDIX
Reading List

Arenson, G. (2001). *Five simple steps to emotional healing.* New York: Fireside.

Callahan, R. J. (2000). *Tapping the healer within using thought field therapy to instantly conquer your fears, anxieties, and emotional distress.* New York: McGraw Hill-NTC.

Flint, G. A. (2001). *Emotional freedom: Techniques for dealing with emotional and physical distress* (Rev. ed.). Vernon, British Columbia. NeoSolTerric Enterprises.

Gallo, F. P. (1998). *Energy psychology: Explorations at the interface of energy, cognition, behavior, and health.* New York: CRC Press.

Gallo, F. P., & Vincenzi, H. (2000). *Energy tapping: How to rapidly eliminate anxiety, depression, cravings, and more using energy psychology.* Oakland, CA: New Harbinger Publications.

Mountrose, P., & Mountrose, J. (1999). *Getting thru to your emotions with EFT: Tap into your hidden potential with the emotional freedom techniques.* Arroyo Grande, CA: Holistic Communications.

Traumatic Incident Reduction:
A Person-Centered, Client-Titrated
Exposure Technique

Frank A. Gerbode

SUMMARY. Traumatic Incident Reduction (TIR) is a person-centered, yet intensely focused approach to trauma resolution, based on the principle that the very act of trying to repress painful memories is what holds them in place and gives them power over the individual. TIR consists of a safe and structured method for reviewing the contents of a past trauma repeatedly at a pace and with a degree of exposure determined by the client. By applying the TIR technique to a traumatic memory in a one-on-one setting with a trained facilitator, the client can discover what he or she needs to know in order to achieve a permanent reduction or elimination of the memory's traumatic aftereffects. *[Article copies available for a fee from The Haworth Document Delivery Service: 1-800- HAWORTH. E-mail address: <docdelivery@haworthpress.com> Website: <http://www.HaworthPress.com> © 2006 by The Haworth Press, Inc. All rights reserved.]*

Address correspondence to Frank A. Gerbode, MD, 650 Adler Court, Sonoma, CA 95476 (E-mail: frank@metapsy.org).

[Haworth co-indexing entry note]: "Traumatic Incident Reduction: A Person-Centered, Client-Titrated Exposure Technique." Gerbode, Frank A. Co-published simultaneously in *Journal of Aggression, Maltreatment & Trauma* (The Haworth Maltreatment & Trauma Press, an imprint of The Haworth Press, Inc.) Vol. 12, No. 1/2, 2006, pp. 151-167; and: *Trauma Treatment Techniques: Innovative Trends* (ed: Jacqueline Garrick, and Mary Beth Williams) The Haworth Maltreatment & Trauma Press, an imprint of The Haworth Press, Inc., 2006, pp. 151-167. Single or multiple copies of this article are available for a fee from The Haworth Document Delivery Service [1-800-HAWORTH, 9:00 a.m. - 5:00 p.m. (EST). E-mail address: docdelivery@haworthpress.com].

KEYWORDS. Person-centered, TIR, Traumatic Incident Reduction, trauma, exposure, PTSD, posttraumatic stress disorder

Traumatic Incident Reduction (TIR; Gerbode, 1989) is a highly structured, person-centered, one-on-one procedure used to reduce or eliminate the negative psychological effects of past traumas and to promote insight and personal growth. In TIR, the client reviews a past traumatic incident repeatedly at her own pace and under the guidance of a trained facilitator until an "end point" (i.e., a point of resolution) is reached. While the client will usually reach an end point in a single session, further work may be required in subsequent sessions on that incident or other associated traumas. For example, it may be necessary for some clients to review earlier, related incidents in order to achieve a full resolution of a given trauma.

Although TIR can be viewed as a form of exposure therapy or deconditioning, the core importance of client insight to the resolution process distinguishes TIR from procedures based mainly on a conditioning model. In addition, TIR differs from the various "energy therapies," such as Thought Field Therapy (TFT) (http://www.tftrx.com), Tapas Acupressure Technique (TAT) (http://www.tat-intl.com), and Eye Movement Desensitization and Reprocessing (EMDR) (Shapiro, 1995), in that it is not explained on the basis of hypothesized, non-experienceable physical or paraphysical entities or processes (e.g., energy flows, meridians, or neural networks). Rather, TIR is based only on experience common to and recognizable by everyone, such as memories, feelings, and thoughts.

TIR is based on an experiential discipline named "metapsychology." Freud (1896/1966) used "metapsychology" to refer to the theory that underlay the practice of psychoanalysis. Freud's term has been updated to mean the careful definition, study, classification, and analysis of those common and universal elements of human experience that anyone, including clients and therapists, can easily recognize. While parapsychology and metaphysics concern themselves with uncommon experiences, metapsychology deals with what is common in experience. Thus, it can form a basis for agreement and understanding, and can serve as a secure base for any experiential or person-centered psychological system. All terms used in metapsychology are carefully and precisely defined and denote things that anyone can directly experience. Thus, the terminology and principles of metapsychology are clear and easy to grasp intuitively.

The reader can verify or falsify each assertion made in metapsychology simply by consulting her own personal experience.

Metapsychology was conceived by this author as a way of being person-centered and, at the same time, directive and structured. While we believe Carl Rogers' person-centered approach (Rogers, 1951) is essential in creating a safe therapeutic environment, we also believe that the focus provided by a structured and directive approach can greatly speed up the process of trauma resolution and other positive changes.

The challenge in addressing this limitation of person-centered treatment approaches thus involves determining the best way to provide clients with structure without imposing a belief system on them. Metapsychology meets this challenge, in that the therapist can structure the session while referring only to metapsychology-based elements that the client already knows to be part of his experience. In that way, the session structure does not impose anything foreign on the client. For instance, one can speak much more safely about memories, feelings, and thoughts than about archetypes, castration anxiety, and the id.

Metapsychology was derived, in part, from the philosophical studies of this author, who first encountered the idea of a science of experience when reading Edmund Husserl (1977). Metapsychology can be viewed as an extension and clarification of Husserl's work. Many of the ideas about how people universally construct their experience were derived from Nelson Goodman (1978) and Michael Polanyi (1962). The methods of linguistic analysis that were highly fashionable in the mid years of this century (Hare, 1952; Moore, 1993) proved a useful anodyne for the turgid prose that seemed to plague Husserl and his fellow phenomenologists. Furthermore, careful attention to terminology has paid off in constructing a clear and consistent taxonomy for metapsychology. This author first encountered the basic concept behind TIR in reading Freud (1910/1984):

> What left the symptom behind was not always a *single* experience. On the contrary, the result was usually brought about by the convergence of several traumas, and often by the repetition of a great number of similar ones. Thus it was necessary to reproduce the whole chain of pathogenic memories in chronological order, or rather in reversed order, the latest ones first and the earliest ones last; and it was quite impossible to jump over the later traumas in order to get back more quickly to the first, which was often the most potent one. (p. 37)

That is a fairly accurate description of the TIR procedure. The work of others, such as Perls (1969), Hubbard (1950), Foa and Rothbaum (1997), Boudewyns and Shipley (1983), Stampfl and Lewis (1967), Beck (1970), and Shapiro (1995), have confirmed the finding that repeatedly addressing a past trauma can resolve it.[1]

In practice, TIR differs from other approaches to trauma by making an unusual combination of two very different elements: (a) complete, person-centered respect for the authority of the client concerning his own experience; and (b) a highly structured, predictable approach that allows both practitioner and client to have a clear understanding of exactly what each is to do and why. Respect for the authority of the client concerning his own experience is incompatible with the quasi-medical model on which some therapies are based. In metapsychology, rather than conceiving of a doctor-like therapist who treats a patient-like client, one instead speaks of a "facilitator" who helps a "viewer" to do what is called "viewing." Viewing, which is the primary activity of a client, consists of the viewer placing his/her awareness on and examining aspects of his/her experience. The facilitator's function is to provide a structure, a safe environment, and a methodology that the viewer can use to discharge the traumas and reach insight. The facilitator does not do anything to the viewer; rather, the viewer has a job to do and the facilitator helps him do it.

WHAT IS TRAUMA?

What makes an experience traumatic? It does not appear to be based entirely on the nature of the incident itself. For example, some Vietnam veterans have been severely traumatized by combat, while others (though probably not the majority) regard it as the high point of their lives or a time when they could demonstrate their best qualities, such as courage and skill. Some have later sought experiences that, like combat, are stimulating and challenging, while others avoid incidents that are similar in any way. Nor is the traumatic nature of an incident entirely inherent in the individual. It is unlikely that a global "resilience" exists that applies to all kinds of challenging events. For example, a person who does not find combat traumatic might easily be traumatized by a significant loss of prestige or by the loss of a loved one. In summary, trauma inheres neither entirely in the challenging experience nor entirely in the experiencer. Trauma is a particular *relationship* between the two, and can be defined as an experience that is of such a quality or intensity that the person having the experience cannot or does not fully confront it while it is happening.

To adopt Freud's terminology, the incident is fully or partially repressed; that is, it remains unexamined and unintegrated into the person's world. Sometimes, the pace of events is too fast to allow the person time to assimilate the experience. For instance, a soldier in the heat of battle needs to keep moving, to keep thinking about and implementing strategies for survival. He cannot afford the luxury of sitting down quietly and contemplating the experience and what it all means. In addition, the experience may be too shocking or painful to confront easily, so he tries to mentally turn away from it (i.e., repress it).

Trauma and its attendant repression always involves an element of procrastination. The person blocks the act of becoming fully aware of and integrating the experience and puts it off until later. It then remains as an incomplete task. Such "unfinished business" has two principle negative effects on an individual. First, it ties up some of his/her mental energy, so that less is available to place on other matters. Hence, the person may be somewhat listless and unenergetic in life. Second, the repressed material lies just below awareness and can easily begin to be brought to mind ("triggered") by the presence of thoughts, feelings, or perceptions that are similar to those contained in the trauma, as a kind of Pavlovian "conditioned reflex" (Pavlov, 1927). When this happens, she experiences a partial or complete reliving of the trauma. Sometimes she is aware of the trauma that has been triggered, but often she is only aware that she is having uncomfortable thoughts, feelings, or perceptions.

The energy drain is an unmitigated liability to the person. While the triggering effect appears to be a liability, it can also be seen as an opportunity. If, after a trauma has been brought to mind ("triggered"), the person has an opportunity to examine it systematically at her own pace in a safe environment, then she can seize the opportunity, complete the process of awareness and integration that was procrastinated, recover the energy that was tied up in the trauma, and return more fully into the here and now, more able to take on other tasks. On the other hand, if she fails to take the opportunity, the triggering becomes a liability because the result is the creation of another trauma. The triggering causes pain by bringing to mind some of the painful contents of the original trauma. If the person shies away from the pain instead of confronting it, then, by the above definition of trauma, she creates another trauma. Thus, there is now a sequence of two traumas containing similar feelings and having some similarities of subject matter, the later one secondary to the earlier. The first trauma is termed the "root" of the sequence, and the second one a "sequent." The content of the sequent is now added to that of the root, and events containing stimuli similar to stimuli in the sequent can trigger both traumas, even if these stimuli do not occur in the root. Thus, further triggerings occur more easily and more frequently, until there can be a large number of traumas in the sequence. As the number of sequents increases, it becomes easier and easier for another triggering to occur and for another traumatic sequent to be created. The person experiences increasing levels of discomfort in different kinds of situations, until she may eventually reach a point of being continually triggered, constantly feeling the pain and constantly repressing it.

To make matters worse, there may be more than one sequence of traumas, each leading back to its own root. Some incidents contained in one sequence may also be contained in others, so that the eventual picture is that of a number of crisscrossing sequences, forming a network of traumatic incidents, called the "traumatic incident network" or "net" (see Figure 1). A person with many heavily charged sequences forming a dense net will have many of the symptoms of posttraumatic stress disorder (PTSD). The net exists, however, in virtually everyone. Almost everyone has some past traumas that have not been fully addressed. This is part of the human condition. Fortunately, it is one that we can do something about, and in so doing we can learn and grow stronger.

The TIR Protocol

In following the TIR protocol, the viewer does what he needs to do to confront a traumatic incident fully. What does it take to confront an in-

FIGURE 1. The Traumatic Incident Network (Net)

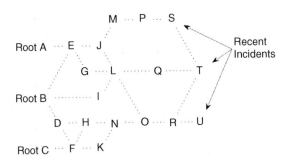

cident? An incident is not like a snapshot that can be taken in at a glance, nor is it like a slide show. Rather, it is like a motion picture, only with other perceptions added to sight and sound. It has a time dimension: a beginning, a definite sequence of events, and an end. To fully familiarize yourself with a movie, you need to actually watch it from beginning to end, at a reasonable speed and in proper chronological sequence without any gaps. To become even more familiar with it, it can be watched repeatedly, with the viewer learning from each viewing. Furthermore, one's understanding of the movie will benefit from reflecting on it and discussing it with friends. However, it is important that the act of watching the movie be separate from that of thinking or talking about it. While watching, you are in a receptive mode. While thinking or talking, you are in an integrative mode, digesting the data obtained from your observations. Both modes are important, but they cannot be done at the same time. For instance, one cannot effectively listen and talk simultaneously. We are simply not built that way. This explains why conventional therapy does not work well for treating trauma. When you watch a critique of a film on television, where there is a great deal of commentary and little contact with the actual film, you do not gain true knowledge and appreciation of the film. You have to watch the film itself. Similarly, briefly contacting a trauma and then spending a great deal of time talking about it does not permit the close examination of the entire incident that is needed for its resolution.

In the TIR technique, therefore, experiential contact with the incident is temporally separated from the cognitive processing that happens after the incident is viewed. The viewer "runs" the incident silently, like a videotape, then talks about it, then runs it again, then talks about it, and so on, until he reaches the end point.

TIR IN DETAIL

The first step in the TIR protocol is an appraisal that the facilitator and viewer make together to determine which traumatic incident to address first. The question of what to work on and in what order is non-trivial. Some incidents that might, on the surface, appear traumatic are not actually so. The viewer may have confronted them fully when they happened, so that no repression occurred and the incidents pose no problems now. Addressing such an "uncharged" incident can actually have serious consequences, since, paradoxically enough, trying to resolve something that is not actually a problem can be very upsetting.

The issue will never go away, because it was not there as a problem in the first place! For example, as a teenager, one Vietnam veteran discovered the body of his mother, who had committed suicide by hanging herself. Later, he joined the military for a double tour of duty, after which he began to suffer from nightmares, hypervigilance, and flashbacks about his Vietnam experiences. During a long course of psychotherapy, therapists repeatedly told him he needed to "work through" the incident of the suicide. He kept working on it, but it never seemed to resolve. Later, in a TIR session, he discovered that the incident had never carried any significant charge for him. It came as a considerable relief to him when his facilitator accepted the fact that it was uncharged and did not need to be addressed.

Some incidents, though highly charged (or, rather, because they are so highly charged) are not yet available for reviewing, because they are too deeply buried and, if brought to consciousness, would overwhelm the viewer. The concept of an "awareness threshold" is useful, here (see Figure 2). The awareness threshold is the dividing line between those incidents that are readily accessible to consciousness and those that are not. Incidents above the threshold are entirely uncharged and unrepressed; that is, they are ordinary data that is not perfectly, but adequately, remembered. Those incidents below the threshold are wholly or partly repressed and, therefore, traumatic. The facilitator is not trying

FIGURE 2. The Awareness Threshold

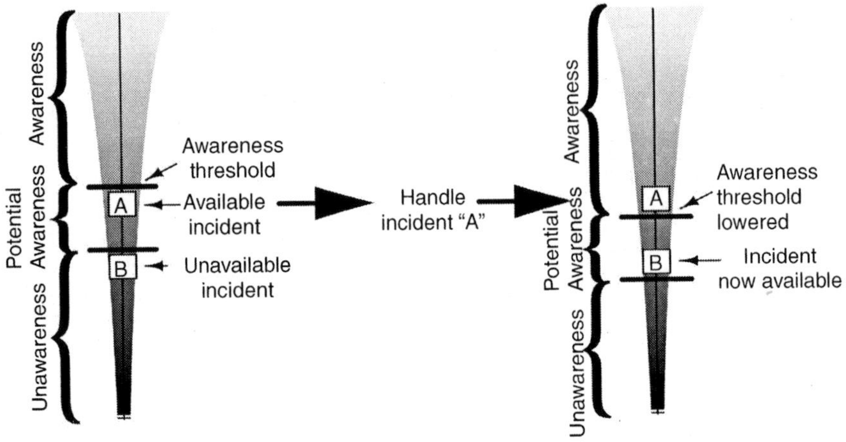

to handle incidents that are uncharged (i.e., above the threshold; e.g., Incident A) or too heavily charged (i.e., too far below it; e.g., Incident C). Instead, she is targeting incidents that lie just below the awareness threshold (e.g., Incident B). When the viewer has taken up and resolved Incident B, it then lies above the awareness threshold, since it has been unrepressed and discharged. Effectively, too, the awareness threshold is lowered. Now Incident C, which before was too deeply buried, enters the zone of potential awareness, and the viewer can fruitfully address it with TIR. Eventually, the viewer brings to light and resolves all incidents that had previously been too deeply buried, and at that point, she is done with TIR. She also no longer carries the diagnosis of PTSD.

How can facilitator and viewer tell when an incident is close to the surface? The key is the viewer's interest. He feels attracted to it, interested in it. He knows intuitively there is something to be gained from looking at the incident and wants to look at it. In choosing an incident to run, then, the facilitator has the viewer make a list of traumas and asks him which is most interesting or which seems to attract his attention the most; the incident the viewer identifies is the one to start with. After completing TIR by reviewing the first identified incident to an end point, the facilitator checks whether the viewer is interested in any other traumas and, if so, which is now the most interesting. That incident is subsequently addressed in turn. Eventually, the viewer no longer feels that it is interesting or necessary to look at any more traumas, because there is no more charge on any of them.[2] At that point, he has completed TIR.

THE STEPS OF TIR

Having found something to work on, one uses seven different instructions in a set pattern to structure the viewer's approach to addressing the traumatic incident.

When

The first step of working on a traumatic incident is to ask when it happened. The viewer can answer with as much or as little precision as he wishes. The facilitator accepts whatever he says without comment. The purpose of this step is twofold. First, a traumatic incident has a way of floating in time, so that, though repressed, it paradoxically seems perpetually to pervade the viewer's here-and-now. Asking when it happened requires the viewer to see the incident in its proper temporal context. Establishing the temporal distance between now and then helps to give the viewer a good perspective from which to view the incident. He can see it better when looking at it from the outside instead of being embedded in it. Second, asking "when" helps the viewer settle upon a *specific* incident that happened at a *particular* time. Otherwise, the viewer might try to run something that is not an incident but a generality, such as "being emotionally abused as a child;" alternatively, he may try to run a series of incidents all at the same time. Having the viewer confront one incident at a time is much easier on him.

Where

For similar reasons, one asks where the incident happened. Any degree of precision is acceptable.

Length

The facilitator then asks how long the incident lasts. Again, whatever the viewer says is acceptable, so long as it is clear that he is talking about one specific incident, not a generality or a series of incidents. The viewer should not confuse the aftermath of an incident, in which the incident may be repeatedly triggered, with the incident itself, which is much briefer. Most traumas last only minutes, rarely hours, and very rarely days.

Begin

Next, the facilitator asks the viewer to "rewind the videotape" by having him go to the starting point of the incident. He is to inform the facilitator when he arrives there, so the facilitator will know when to give the next instruction. The starting point is usually the first point at which the viewer had some inkling that something bad was going to happen. Sometimes, he needs to start even a little earlier, because the principal trauma may have consisted of the shocking contrast between the pleasant time preceding the trauma and the trauma itself.

Aware

The viewer next says what he is aware of at the exact starting point of the incident. The viewer should achieve a "freeze frame" at that point, with no action in it. This step helps establish for facilitator and viewer what the starting point is. It also helps the viewer gain mastery over the unrolling of the incident, which, when previously triggered, always moved forward on its own.

Go

The next step is for the viewer to go through to the end of the incident. He should do so silently, as explained above. Some viewers cannot seem to remain silent while running an incident. If they need to talk, that is acceptable. Later, they will probably be able to confront running through incidents silently.

Tell

Next, the facilitator asks the viewer to articulate what happened. This is an open-ended question. On this step, the facilitator listens without comment to whatever the viewer has to say until he is done. The viewer may relate the contents of the incident, talk about the reactions and feelings he had when running through it, or express any thoughts he may have about the incident or about anything else. This step completes the first time through the incident. Four of the above steps (when, where, length, aware) are orientation steps and are not repeated on subsequent runs; begin, go, and tell are used for all but the first run.

THE PATTERN OF A TIR SESSION

As the viewer goes through the incident several times, he will most likely manifest a marked change in his affect (see Figure 3). Typically, the viewer starts at a moderate level of affect and begins to display more and more affect on subsequent runs, until the affect reaches a peak, then begins to diminish in intensity until it plateaus at or near zero and the viewer achieves an end point. There are three cardinal signs of an end point: positive indicators, extroversion, and realizations. With regard to positive indicators, an end point is always accompanied by an improvement in the viewer's affect. The viewer feels relieved, serene, cheerful, or even enthusiastic or exhilarated. If the viewer still appears glum or otherwise stuck in some uncomfortable emotion, he has not reached an end point. In addition, until a viewer has resolved an incident, his attention is fixed upon it. He is trying to look at it, to figure it out, to deal with

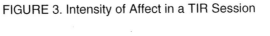

FIGURE 3. Intensity of Affect in a TIR Session

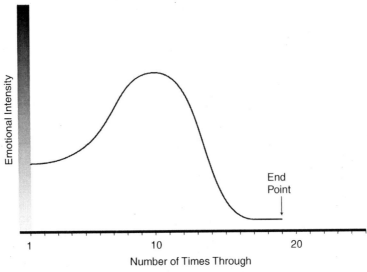

it in some way. At an end point, the viewer's attention is freed from the task of viewing and considering the incident. He shows this by visibly appearing more present. If his eyes were shut, he opens them. He looks around or makes some kind of comment indicating that he is back in touch with the here and now and is no longer fixated on the incident; thus the viewer exhibits more extroversion. Finally, the viewer who reaches the end point will often come up with insights and realizations about himself, others, life, or any other topic spontaneously. The content of the realization does not matter. What is important is that the viewer has had the subjective experience of having realized something. Positive indicators and extroversion are both necessary and sufficient conditions of the viewer's having attained an end point in TIR; realization is a good corroborating point but is not always present. Deciding when an end point has occurred is the most important judgment call the facilitator will have to make. Fortunately, with practice, end points are easy to spot.

When the facilitator observes what appears to be an end point, she asks the viewer whether this seems to be a good point at which to end the session. If he says, "Yes," the therapist informs him that the session is ended. There is no rehashing, summarizing, or commenting in any way on what has happened in the session. Letting the viewer take his success and go home with it, without further ado, is quite empowering to him. If the facilitator engages in or encourages any post-viewing inquiry about or discussion of the resolved incident, she risks invalidating the viewer's end point.

EARLIER INCIDENTS

About half the time, a TIR session follows a somewhat different pattern. After the affect peaks and begins to drop, it then levels out short of going to zero and remains unchanged for several runs. At the same time, the viewer will be telling more or less the same story on the Tell step. When this pattern appears, there is probably an earlier, related incident on the traumatic sequence, or possibly the current incident starts earlier. Though the current incident itself may have trauma-inducing contents, some significant part of the pain in the incident comes from an incident earlier in the sequence or from an earlier part of the current incident.

At this point, it is necessary first to check whether there is an earlier starting point for the incident. If so, the facilitator asks the viewer to go to the new starting point and tell her when he gets there. TIR then continues from the Aware step. If there is no earlier beginning, it is necessary to check for an earlier and similar incident. Usually, the viewer will find an incident sitting right at the edge of consciousness. The TIR procedure is then repeated, including When, Where, etc., exactly as given above, to an end point or (sometimes) to a point where, again, it is necessary to go earlier. In practice, one rarely has to go earlier more than once or twice before reaching the root incident, and then an end point appears. In fact, it is only because of the end point indicators that one can tell that the viewer has reached the root. It is both necessary and sufficient to reach and resolve the root in order to discharge the entire sequence.

By now, the reader will have guessed that running a traumatic incident or sequence, which almost always should be done in one session, requires some flexibility in session length. Sessions may run anywhere from one to four hours. An average session length is 1 1/2 hours, and it is fairly rare to see sessions going on for more than 2 1/2 hours. Some viewers who are just starting TIR or addressing particularly heavy incidents sometimes require three or (rarely) four hours to reach an end point. The flexibility required for TIR poses some practical difficulties, but these can be overcome. With a new viewer, it is best to schedule him as the last client of the day to avoid worrying about time constraints.

CREATING A SAFE ENVIRONMENT

Running traumatic incidents is hard work for the viewer, who is finally confronting issues he has probably avoided for years. In order to do so, he needs to feel safe enough to devote all of his attention to the incident(s) he is running. It does not work for him to have some of his attention absorbed by worrying about the process of the session or about what the facilitator might think, say, or do. The facilitator alleviates worries about the structure and process of the session by explaining the TIR procedure in detail to the viewer, so he knows precisely what the facilitator is going to say during the session. Since TIR is repetitive and predictable, the process tends to fade into the background, which is as it should be.

Part of the facilitator's modus operandi consists of a series of strict rules, the intent of which is to produce a safe session environment by establishing a suitable division of labor between facilitator and viewer. The facilitator is in charge of maintaining the structure of the session and determining its process. The viewer is the one who actually does all the steps and is the authority on the content of what he views and its meaning. The facilitator acts like a good secretary and treats the viewer as an executive. A secretary keeps things organized and handles appointments and the structure of the executive's day, while the executive actively does the most vital functions, which in this case are viewing and attaining insights and personal growth.

The most important rule is not, under any circumstances, to make any assertions, suggestions, or evaluations of any kind to the viewer about oneself, the viewer, or anything the viewer has said or done. The focus is on being interested in the viewer, and not interesting to him. Exercises in applying these rules consistently in a TIR session form an important part of the TIR training.

Another crucial part of the training consists of communication exercises that refine some micro-skills needed to run TIR effectively. These exercises enhance the ability to be present fully to a viewer, regardless of what he is saying or doing. They reduce the possibility of burnout by helping keep one's attention extroverted on the viewer rather than introverted upon oneself. Since the communication exercises require time under close supervision to overcome old habits, and because TIR has some complexities in its application that are beyond the scope of this article, it is essential to receive the full, official training in TIR under the supervision of a qualified TIR trainer in order to obtain consistently good results from using the procedure.

CASE EXAMPLE

Pete was a 33-year-old man who complained of anxiety, intrusive thoughts, marital problems, and hypervigilance following a gang-related beating. He had had no PTSD symptoms before the beating. In the first of three sessions, he did Unblocking (a TIR-related technique) on the incident. In the second, he addressed "feeling embarrassed" as a theme for TIR. In the third and final session, he addressed the incident itself with TIR, to a good end point. At that point, his PTSD symptoms disappeared and had not returned on follow-up four years later. The total time elapsed in the three sessions was 6 hours 23 minutes.

RESEARCH ON TIR

TIR has been shown to be effective in two controlled outcome studies. In one (Valentine, 1997), TIR was found to be significantly better than no treatment on the Posttraumatic Symptom Scale (PSS), The Beck Depression Inventory (BDI), the Clinical Anxiety Scale (CAS), and the Generalized Expectancy of Success Scale (GESS). In the other (Bisbey, 1995), TIR was found significantly better than controls and also significantly better than Direct Therapeutic Exposure for the same period of treatment time (an average of 16.5 hours), as measured by the Penn Inventory, Impact of Event Scale, Crime-Related PTSD Scale, and the Individual Trauma Checklist. Qualitative studies on TIR also suggest that TIR is effective (Carbonell & Figley, 1995, 1996; Coughlin, 1995; Valentine, 2000; Valentine & Smith, 2001). None of the studies done on TIR has shown or suggested that it is not effective.

FUTURE AREAS OF APPLICATION

There are certain populations for whom TIR does not work well, as currently formulated. Young children, for instance, often do not have sufficient interest and power of concentration to stay focused on a traumatic incident long enough to resolve it. The "Conversational Remedy"

(Gerbode, 1989, p. 548), a shortened and simplified form of TIR, can be used with some children, although in cases of severe trauma it is unlikely to be sufficient. It would be interesting to see if the principles and overall pattern of TIR could be incorporated into a play therapy session of some kind to keep the child engaged while repeatedly reviewing an incident. Such a technique could also be applied to selected adults.

For a variety of reasons, some adults are not ready to do TIR. A number of metapsychology-based techniques can be useful to bring a client to a point of readiness. These methods are somewhat complex and require a fair amount of training and experience. It would be helpful to find ways to simplify and standardize these preparatory steps.

TIR-like techniques, which embody a very highly structured, yet strictly person-centered approach, are also useful for addressing non-trauma-related issues, such as self-esteem issues, relationship problems, and work and career related problems. At this writing, many such techniques are available and are in the process of being systematized into a brief, easy-to-learn format.

NOTES

1. For more data on the background of TIR and its relationship to other procedures, see Robert Moore's excellent article on the World Wide Web (http://www.tir.org/metapsy/psychfnd.htm).

2. The principle of following the viewer's interest is part of all metapsychology-based viewing techniques. An interesting result of taking this approach is that you will not encounter "resistance" in your clients. Resistance occurs when the client does not want to take a course of action that the therapist feels is necessary.

REFERENCES

Beck, A. T. (1970). Role of fantasies in psychotherapy and psychopathology. *The Journal of Nervous and Mental Disease, 150,* 3-17.

Bisbey, L. B. (1995). *No longer a victim: A treatment outcome study of crime victims with post-traumatic stress disorder.* Unpublished doctoral dissertation, California School of Professional Psychology, San Diego, CA.

Boudewyns, P. A., & Shipley, R. H. (1983). *Flooding and implosive therapy: Direct therapeutic exposure in clinical practice.* New York: Plenum Publishing Corporation.

Carbonell, J., & Figley, C. (1995). *The active ingredient project: Initial findings.* Unpublished manuscript.

Carbonell, J., & Figley, C. (1996). A systematic clinical demonstration methodology: A collaboration between practitioners and clinical researchers. *The Traumatology Forum, 2* (1), Article 1. Available from, <http://www.fsu.edu/~trauma/art1v2i1.html>.

Coughlin, W. E. (1995). *Traumatic incident reduction: Efficacy in treating anxiety symptomatology.* Unpublished doctoral dissertation, Union University, Jackson, TN.

Foa, E. B., & Rothbaum, B. O. (1997). *Treating the trauma of rape.* New York: Guilford Publications.

Freud, S. (1966). Letter to Wilhelm Fliess. In J. Strachey (Ed. & Trans.), *The standard edition of the complete psychological works of Sigmund Freud* (Vol. 1, p. 274). London: Hogarth Press. (Original work published 1896.)

Freud, S. (1984). *Two short accounts of psycho-analysis* J. Strachey (Ed. & Trans.), (p. 37). Singapore: Penguin Books. (Original work published 1910.)

Gerbode, F. A. (1989). *Beyond psychology: An introduction to metapsychology.* Kansas City, MO: TIRA Press.

Goodman, N. (1978). *Ways of world making.* Indianapolis, IN: Hackett Publishing Co, Inc

Hare, R. M. (1952). *The language of morals.* Oxford: Oxford University Press.

Hubbard, L. R. (1950) *Dianetics, the modern science of mental health.* New York: Hermitage House Publishing.

Husserl, E. (1977). *Cartesian meditations.* Dordrecht, Netherlands: Kluwer Academic Publishers.

Moore, G. E. (1903). *Principia ethica.* Cambridge: Cambridge University Press.

Moore, R. H. (1993). Traumatic incident reduction: A cognitive-emotive treatment of post-traumatic stress disorder. In W. Dryden & L. Hill (Eds.), *Innovations in rational-emotive therapy* (pp. 116-159). Newbury Park, CA: Sage.

Pavlov, I. P. (1927). *Conditioned reflexes.* New York: Oxford University Press.

Perls, F. (1969). *Gestalt therapy.* New York: Julian Press.

Polanyi, M. (1962). *Personal knowledge.* London: Routledge and Kegan Paul.

Rogers, C. (1951). *Client-centered therapy.* Boston, MA: Houghton Mifflin.

Shapiro, F. (1995) *Eye movement desensitization and reprocessing.* New York: Guilford Press.

Stampfl, T. G., & Lewis, D. J. (1967). Essentials of implosive therapy: A learning-theory-based psychodynamic behavioral therapy. *Journal of Abnormal Psychology, 72,* 496-503.

Valentine, P. V. (1997). *Traumatic incident reduction: Brief treatment of trauma-related symptoms in incarcerated females.* Unpublished doctoral dissertation, Florida State University.

Valentine, P. V. (2000) Traumatic Incident Reduction I: Traumatized women inmates: Particulars of practice and research. *Journal of Offender Rehabilitation, 31*(3-4), 1-15.

Valentine, P. V., & Smith, T. E. (2001). Evaluating Traumatic Incident Reduction (TIR) therapy with female inmates: A randomized controlled clinical trial. *Research on Social Work Practice, 11*(1), 40-52.

The Humor of Trauma Survivors: Its Application in a Therapeutic Milieu

Jacqueline Garrick

SUMMARY. This article focuses on how the sense of humor that trauma survivors have can be used to assist them in mitigating the intensity of their traumatic stress reactions. A brief review of the literature on the nature of humor and its ability to diffuse stressful situations and reactions is provided. It is suggested that despite the fact that humor is often underappreciated and ignored in the therapeutic process, it can actually be a powerful healing tool when both the therapist and the client are willing to openly discuss it. Humor does not minimize the significance of a terrible event, but it does allow the survivor to see how they can cope and thrive in their environment. *[Article copies available for a fee from The Haworth Document Delivery Service: 1-800-HAWORTH. E-mail address: <docdelivery@haworthpress.com> Website: <http://www.HaworthPress.com> © 2006 by The Haworth Press, Inc. All rights reserved.]*

KEYWORDS. Trauma, survivor, sense of humor, black humor, gallows humor

---

Address correspondence to Jacqueline Garrick, 2 Narrows Court, Silver Spring, MD 20906 (Email: cptjax@aol.com).

[Haworth co-indexing entry note]: "The Humor of Trauma Survivors: Its Application in a Therapeutic Milieu." Garrick, Jacqueline. Co-published simultaneously in *Journal of Aggression, Maltreatment & Trauma* (The Haworth Maltreatment & Trauma Press, an imprint of The Haworth Press, Inc.) Vol. 12, No. 1/2, 2006, pp. 169-182; and: *Trauma Treatment Techniques: Innovative Trends* (ed: Jacqueline Garrick, and Mary Beth Williams) The Haworth Maltreatment & Trauma Press, an imprint of The Haworth Press, Inc., 2006, pp. 169-182. Single or multiple copies of this article are available for a fee from The Haworth Document Delivery Service [1-800-HAWORTH, 9:00 a.m. - 5:00 p.m. (EST). E-mail address: docdelivery@haworthpress.com].

Available online at http://www.haworthpress.com/web/JAMT
doi:10.1300/J146v12n01_09

Many years ago, while counseling a Vietnam veteran, we entered into a discussion on what he did for fun. He had a great deal of difficulty identifying anything that was fun for him and finally said, "I go to work." This brief exchange led to a journey of understanding the usefulness of humor as a therapeutic tool when confronting traumatic experiences in therapy. Upon researching this issue and its application in individual and group settings, this author discovered a book entitled, *Laughter in Hell: The Use of Humor During the Holocaust* (Lipman, 1991), which is a collection of humorous anecdotes and jokes told by Holocaust survivors. The fact that Holocaust survivors could use humor to face their plight and their torturers suggests that other trauma survivors could be encouraged to do the same.

Consequently, I introduced this concept in the individual and group therapy that I provided to Vietnam veterans. In therapy, veterans were encouraged to tell funny or ironic stories that helped them get through their tour of duty, as well as the childhood memories that kept their spirits up while in Vietnam. In a group session, for example, one veteran recalled that while his platoon was crossing a rice paddy and he had stopped to fill his canteen with the murky delta water, his mother's childhood warning not to play in mud puddles had come to mind. Other members of the group were also able to recall parental admonishments that, when applied to their experiences in the Vietnam War, seemed absurd. The use of humor was found to assist veterans in developing and recognizing their own brand of humor and in appreciating its healing effects.

The sharing of humorous memories was also found to facilitate group bonding and provide participants with a new perspective for viewing the memories that haunted them. In addition, the humorous exchanges created a safe, comfortable atmosphere in which other more conflicted emotions and memories could be shared with greater ease by providing moments of release when the tension became too great. This author also found that as veterans brought their previously disturbing memories to the surface, integrating their traumatic experiences became easier when the memories were no longer as awful as they had once seemed.

Based on these observations, the use of humor appears to be a beneficial addition to the treatment of trauma survivors. Further support for this notion was provided by Curtis (2001), who found that the use of "humor in support groups promotes cohesiveness, creative problem-solving skills and humanizes the healing process" (p. 7). Due to these benefits, Curtis described humor as a key factor in conducting individual or group debriefings.

The research on humor has indicated that it may be a useful addition to the treatment of a variety of populations. Ellis and Abrams (1994), for example, described the effects of using humor with Rational-Emotive Behavior Therapy (REBT) in the treatment of terminally ill patients. Ellis and Abrams advocate REBT as a way to "reduce irrational beliefs to absurdity, to laugh at them and to see how ironic it is that a presumably sensible person keeps holding onto self-destructive notions" (p. 190). Similarly, in his work with terminally ill patients, Tobin (1999) used humor to help patients find peace with dying. According to Tobin, "addressing fears of dying and long-repressed emotions is a significant turning point in the dying process because it allows you to proceed from the early phases of fear and grasping toward healing and serenity" (p. 52). In a case example, he described a patient who was able to use laughter as a "powerful tool for confronting and lessening his worry" (p. 52) to illustrate this point.

Tobin's (1999) approach could be considered congruent with cognitive-behavioral therapy in that it seeks to correct "the pathological elements of the fear structure" (Foa, Keane & Friedman, 2000, p. 61). Rothbaum, Meadows, Resick, and Foy (cited in Foa et al.) claimed that it does this by first activating the pathological fear structures and then by providing new information "that includes elements that are incompatible with the existing pathological elements so that they can be corrected" (p. 61). There are several cognitive-behavioral techniques reviewed by Rothbaum et al., including Stress Inoculation Training (SIT), which incorporates education, relaxation, breathing exercises, and self-dialog. Friedman (2000) defines SIT as "a variety of anxiety management techniques designed to increase coping skills for current situations" (p. 45). The use of humor can be viewed as a component of SIT that acts as a conduit when therapists are working with clients towards integrating corrective information and modifying pathological components of traumatizing memories, as demonstrated by Tobin's work with the terminally ill.

Additionally, the literature on humor supports the notion that humor has the physiological and psychological ability to promote healing (Fry & Salameh, 1987). The ability to tap into the body's own "anti-depressants" is an important factor to consider when providing therapy. Therefore, understanding our neurological responses to laughter and general happiness, as well as the nature of humor, represents an asset to therapy.

NEUROPHYSIOLOGY AND HUMOR

Why does it feel so good to laugh? When a person laughs, the pituitary gland produces hormones called endorphins, which act as natural pain killers. Endorphins, when released into the system, create an effect similar to taking morphine, heroin, or some other type of opiate (Berk, 1994). Therefore, people who are "high on life" are often thought to be experiencing the effects of these hormones. This is similar to the "adrenaline rushes" described by athletes when they increase their heart rate and feel euphoric. Cousins (1979), in his classic book, *Anatomy of an Illness*, claimed that viewing comedic movies prior to going to bed at night represents a way to decrease his pain level and allow him to get restful restorative sleep without the use of sleep medication.

According to Keith-Spiegal, "laughter and humor have been hailed as good for the body because they restore homeostasis, stabilize blood pressure, oxygenate the blood, massage vital organs, stimulate circulation, facilitate digestion, relax the system, and produce feelings of well-being" (Fry & Salameh, 1987, p. 11). When oxygen is flowing better, the respiratory system benefits, resulting in less yawning and lower levels of sleepiness. Once endorphins have been released and blood is flowing to the brain and muscles, individuals begin to feel better, have more energy, and feel less stressed. Concentration also becomes easier and tasks can be completed quicker as basic levels of functioning improve.

Researchers have also found evidence that mirthful laughter can increase the body's ability to fight infection. For example, Berk (1994) showed that there were five significant neuroendocrine and stress hormone changes that occur during laughter. First, laughter was found to cause an increase in the number of one's activated T cells (T lymphocytes), which leads to an activation of the immune system. Second, an increase in the T cells with the receptors that neurotransmitters connect to also occurs with laughter. Third, laughter was found to produce an increase in natural killer cells, which fight viral infections and cancer cells. Berk's findings also demonstrated an increase in immunoglobulin A antibodies in the upper respiratory tract during laughter, which allows this system to fight infection. Finally, the study found the levels of gamma interferon, one of the cytokines of the immune system responsible for activating the immune system, also increase during laughter. Berk also noted that laughter has been suggested to be responsible for increasing interleukin-2, which also boosts immunity. Additional research, however, is needed in this area for scientists to understand the psychophysiological and psychoneuroimmunological effects of humor and laughter on the body better.

UNDERSTANDING HUMOR

Generally, many clients enter therapy to achieve the common goal of finding a sense of happiness. Survivors of abuse, crime, disaster, and war often seek out therapy for this basic reason. Traditional psychotherapy assumes that the way to happiness is to restore the client's self-esteem or self-worth.

Humor is a human trait that is often summoned to combat a stressful situation, whether it be to enhance a sense of belonging in a social situation (i.e., "the life of the party" or the "class clown") or to diffuse tension. It is the component of human nature that helps make concepts and experiences seem amusing or comical. Fun, according to Patch Adams (1993) is "humor in action" (p. 66). Having a good sense of humor is a valued trait in our society. Humor often leads to forgiveness and letting go of worries. Ellis and Abrams (1994) described it as being connected to the ability to view the world as something other than an awful place.

Stress is a normal part of daily life. How one reacts to and handles stress, however, determines how an individual functions in various circumstances. According to Valent (cited in Figley, 1995), "stress responses may be adaptive or maladaptive" (p. 30). Maladaptive responses to stress create distress, while adaptive responses bring eustress. Eustress equates to motivation, competition, and determination, which are important ingredients for success. Consequently, eustress is not only normal, but is also healthy.

According to Figley (1995), Valent's review of survival strategies led him to identify the significance of attachment and conclude that "the emotions of separation and abandonment may be processed by parts of the hypothalamus and the cingulate gyrus" (p. 34). These emotions may also be associated with low levels of opiates. The administration of opiates, for example, reliably suppressed the crying out (distress vocalizations) behaviors caused by separation in all species tested by Pankseep, Meeker, and Bean (cited in Figley, 1995). Since human beings produce their own opiate-like hormone (i.e., endorphins) during laughter, a similar decrease in the level of distress experienced is likely to occur with the introduction of humor and laughter. Very often, the key to stress management, therefore, involves humor. Distress can become eustress when humor is added to a situation. Tension and anxiety can immediately be relieved by a smile or a laugh.

Even children understand that "acting silly" helps them to avoid an unpleasant situation (e.g., punishment). Adults often try to scold a child for a previous negative behavior while they simultaneously laugh at it. Children who act "silly" find that the attention they get from their peers and adults is rewarding, thereby reinforcing its repetition. They learn that it feels good to make other people laugh. Abused children very often use humor to cover up the violence that is being perpetrated in their homes.

Traumatic events and experiences are by no means funny, nor should they be. However, in many cases, survivors and the providers who work with them have used humor to help cope with trauma. For example, a Native American therapist, while discussing poverty and the high rate of chronic illness on the reservation, once joked that their problems resulted from General Custer stopping at the Bureau of Indian Affairs and saying, "Don't do anything until I get back." This quip does not lessen the severity of the problems being discussed, but it does give voice to the frustrations that Native Americans face in dealing with the government. The importance of this humor tactic will be discussed further.

When treating trauma survivors, it is important to understand the nature of their humor. When recalling traumatic memories, humorous instances and acts are often left out of the counseling session due to the fear that the use of humor would be considered disrespectful to the dead and/or injured. Thus, even though humor can help survivors see that there are still pleasures in life despite the tragedy that occurred and, therefore, can be an important part of the healing process, it is still sometimes seen as taboo. Adams (1993) observes, "humor is often denied in the adult world. Almost universally in business, religious, medical and academic worlds, humor is denigrated and even condemned. . . . The stress is on seriousness with the implication that humor is inappropriate" (p. 66). However, if therapists allow survivors to continue to perceive the recollection of pleasant memories or expressing humor in therapy to be in bad taste, they are at risk of fostering the survivor's feelings of guilt, shame, and lack of self-worth. Clients, therefore, need to be encouraged to explore their sense of humor as part of SIT and need to know that they are not alone in acknowledging the laughter amidst the horror.

Fry (2000) acknowledges that "there is an extensive and authenticated humor literature from prison camps, from places where hostages are kept and where torture is taking place, from societies under dictatorships like Nazi Germany or Stalinist Russia. There is also a literature regarding the use of humor at times of natural disasters, like earthquakes, hurricanes, floods and fires" (p. 1). Therapists should refer clients to this literature and ask about their mirthful moments and memories or the amusing characters that have helped them cope. Adams suggests that medical professionals also "be open to experimentation and escalate slowly" (p. 69) as they practice using humor. Therapists, for example, can introduce the topic of humor by simply asking their clients what they do for fun. However, in order to more fully address issues of survivor humor, therapists will first need to understand the two predominate forms of humor that occur in the wake of trauma and be able to recognize when its application is inappropriate. Lipman (1991) identified the two common forms of humor used by survivors as gallows humor and black humor.

GALLOWS HUMOR

Gallows humor is most common among police officers, fire fighters, paramedics, and hospital workers who face death and dying every day. Such individuals often describe their "dark" sense of humor as the only way to "get by" while doing their job. Dick explored this phenomenon among law enforcement and EMS personnel who experienced events that were human-caused, life threatening, belief challenging, media attentive, and identifiable (Doka, 1996). She described anhedonia (i.e., the inability to experience pleasure) as one of the typical traumatic reactions among these groups. Since pleasure is often derived from a sense of humor, she concluded that it becomes necessary for first responders (e.g., emergency personnel) and health care professionals to develop and maintain that sense of humor. When death is all around and pain and suffering are a normal part of the day, using humor to cope can be a very healthy skill. For example, at Walter Reed Army Medical Center's Intensive Care Unit, a colorful sign reading "Thoracic Park" was put out at about the same time that the dinosaur movie, *Jurassic Park*, was a hit.

Jewish literature from the Holocaust is filled with examples of gallows humor. Lipman (1991) explored how Jews used humor to survive the ghettos and concentration camps of Nazism. While it is inconceivable that there was anything to laugh at in Eastern Europe during Hitler's reign, life went on, people fell in love, celebrated holidays, raised families, and told jokes about the Nazis. Often, these jokes were recycled from the days of the Cossacks and the Czar. According to Lipman, concentration camp survivors have reported that part of their ability to survive was due to their efforts to keep faith, hope, and humor alive.   .

BLACK HUMOR

Black humor was born in the United States during slavery (Lipman, 1991). Different from gallows humor, survivors who use black humor have typically faced conditions of oppression and prejudice, but not necessarily annihilation. Rather than focusing on death and destruction, black humor tends to focus on the oppressor and the murderer. Slaves created this brand of humor as a passive-aggressive means of circumventing their oppressors without the risk of retaliation. In addition to using black humor, Maya Angelou (1993) noted that "slaves also devised ways of keeping their souls robust and spirits alive in that awful atmosphere" (pp. 101-102) by addressing each other with familial terms and using sweet tones when speaking to each other. According to Lipman (1991), song was also a commonly employed tool for otherwise prohibited communication of feelings and thoughts during slavery.

The Jews of Hitler's Europe also intertwined the use of black humor with gallows humor. Black humor primarily exists when a trauma is man-made or has a known perpetrator (Lipman, 1991). When survivors joke about Hitler, Custer, the Grand Wizard, or an abuser, they utilize a coping skill that releases anxiety, rage, and depression. The use of black humor, therefore, can be seen as a means of allowing negative or maladaptive stress responses to become positive or adaptive and to facilitate survivors' progress in the recovery process. Unlike Lipman, Kuhlman (cited in Fry & Salameh, 1993) does not distinguish between gallows humor and black humor. Kuhlman described gallows humor as, "violating principles usually associated with human meanings and values. . . . It is an in-kind response to an absurd dilemma, a way of being sane in an insane place" (p. 25).

INAPPROPRIATE HUMOR

The crux of a victim's sense of humor is in the nuances of irony and satire that can be healthily exploited for the purpose of survival. Although humor can be used to facilitate therapeutic gains, one's inappropriate use of humor or affect generally indicates that one is trying to avoid one's true feelings (Marcus, 1990). If a client is smiling and joking while reporting a particularly painful childhood memory, it is likely that the client is not sure how close s/he wants to get to the memory and is attempting to obtain distance from the associated emotional pain. This distancing is similar to denial in that it provides for a comfort zone. However, if not properly handled in treatment, such denial impedes the therapeutic process. According to Marcus, when a client laughs after everything s/he says and attributes this behavior to "nervous laughter," low self-esteem and an underlying lack of confidence in one's own thoughts and opinions is indicated.

Marcus (1990) also noted that "smiling just represents a feeble attempt to either hide their true feelings from themselves, and find others or, more radically, that it actually *stands for,* or is the equivalent of, another internally expressed emotion" (p. 427). The therapist needs to address these underlying emotions by sensitively peeling away at the comical mask that covers them. The therapist must also be able to reflect back the inconsistencies between the client's behavior and what is being reported or recalled. The diagnostic significance of inconsistencies between one's affect and content is dependant on the degree and frequency of such inconsistencies. When affect is inappropriate to content on a regular basis, for example, then other diagnoses (e.g., schizophrenia) need to be ruled out.

As mentioned previously, dehumanizing humor is a weapon of the racist. The racist or the oppressor makes fun of what he does not understand or fears, in spite of its negative impact on others. When an abuser treats someone as if he or she is funny or is not to be taken seriously, then the individual is no longer dangerous and frightening. The power balance is altered and the ridiculer gains more control.

In war, the enemy is traditionally dehumanized. It is much easier to kill or maim another human being if s/he is not seen as fully human. If the enemy can be ridiculed, put down, and devalued, then his fate is of less concern. During military training, soldiers are informally exposed to racial slurs and caricatures of past and present enemies in order to make them better able to survive in a combat zone. For many combat veterans, the collusion in dehumanizing the enemy has resulted in shame, guilt, and remorse that needs to be addressed in the therapeutic process (Brende & Parson, 1985). Since these veterans have had a negative experience with using humor, it may often be harder for them to see humor as a positive technique for their own recovery. The therapist's role is to educate veterans or other clients on the different facets and uses of humor and its appropriateness.

The inappropriate use of humor is also present in many violent domestic situations. Hypothetically, in such scenarios, the perpetrator wants to control the victim and does so by verbally abusing her prior to physically assaulting her. By the time he actually strikes her, she has already been demeaned, belittled, and berated. He has made "fun" of her appearance, habits, intelligence, and anything else she cares about to the point that she has become a non-person. The perpetrator has used humor inappropriately to dehumanize the victim in order to make himself feel stronger, more powerful, and more in control of the dynamics within the dyad. He needs to believe in his own sense of power in order to counter his own frail ego. In addition, the victim comes to accept the perpetrator's picture of her because of its sheer repetition and her own poor self-image. He has ridiculed her and she feels ridiculous. Her ability to "fight back" is gone and she begins to believe that she deserves the abusive treatment.

If victims of domestic violence can successfully discover and use their sense of black humor in their recovery process, they can regain their sense of self by seeing the limits of the abuser's power over them or the abusor's ridiculousness. This can be achieved by using the previously mentioned REBT technique developed by Ellis (Ellis & Abrams, 1994) to challenge and re-process the irrational beliefs the abuser has infused into the victim's self-image. Once victims can see the absurdity of the irrational beliefs held about the self and the perpetrator, their feelings of safety and control can be restored. On the other hand, when the abuser is the client, the therapist will need to assist him in recognizing the irrational nature of his beliefs about relationships and in learning the difference between ridicule and humor. Further development of a perpetrator's sense of humor could help him cope in a healthy manner with tension and anger and replace his negative violent reactions with calmer, more socially acceptable behaviors.

APPLICATIONS FOR HUMOR IN THERAPY

How do therapists access humor in the therapeutic process with clients? As Adams (1993) suggested, therapists must initially recognize how important it is to have a sense of humor and be open to seeing humor in themselves and their own lives before they can use it in the therapy process. Then, they must find out what humor means to the individual clients with whom they are working. In the author's experience, veterans and other trauma survivors report seeing themselves as having a "sick sense of humor." They often felt guilty for the things that they found humorous and believed "normal" people would not laugh at or enjoy similar things. Many hospital personnel and rescue workers tell people, "if you were never on the job, you wouldn't understand." Similarly, when combat veterans say things such as, "If you weren't there, you wouldn't understand," they are expressing a sense of alienation and attempting to reject a society that they fear will reject them because of their military experiences. However, therapists can aid veterans in understanding that their sense of humor is very often a vital part of their ability to cope with emotionally stressful, and sometimes horrific, events given their frame of reference. Educating clients about gallows and black humor can help to relieve such feelings of isolation and separateness. When survivors are able to focus on the use of humor in a therapeutic atmosphere, they can then address their feelings of shame and guilt and see humor for what it is: a stress relieving tool. Developing the tool of humor in a therapeutic milieu helps to enable clients to incoporate one form of stress management or SIT into their daily lives.

It can be difficult to get survivors to discuss what they do for fun or what they think is funny, but the therapist should be in tune with the opportunities for interjecting this notion into the therapeutic process as the clients improve their skills for healthy living. As mentioned earlier, the Vietnam veteran who went to work for fun was eventually able to recognize that he had not allowed himself to have fun since he returned from Vietnam and was consequently able to change his pattern of behavior. Initially, he thought it was funny when people did stupid things and got into trouble. Other people always told him his sense of humor was "gross" and "disgusting." However, after several sessions of therapy, which focused on this issue, he was able to recall what he did for fun before the war and some amusing things from his time in the service. With the therapist, he then contracted a plan to spend time in his week purposefully doing something that he enjoyed (e.g., sports, watch a comedy show, or visit a friend). He re-discovered that he enjoyed telling jokes and began to collect a repertoire to tell at work and at the end of the sessions. He was able to make a conscientious decision to be happy rather than mad and depressed all the time. He was then able to handle previously upsetting situations more lightheartedly, by being able to see the absurdity in his own previously enraged reactions in certain situations.

In the case of this veteran, the use of cognitive therapy to explore humor made a dramatic difference in his sense of self and well-being. He was able to dispute irrational beliefs about himself and his sense of humor and use humor as a coping skill in a healthier positive manner. Problems that came up at work and at home no longer infuriated him and he was better able to use his problem-solving skills to deal with these stressful situations.

Thus, it can be very useful for clients to learn how to recognize and appreciate their own sense of humor and how to benefit from it. To help clients better understand their own sense of humor, the therapist should first have them list the things that they enjoy (or that they once enjoyed) and that help them to relax. When they are under stress, these items become a healthy behavior plan upon which to rely rather than relying on the negative reactions that have previously made their situation worse. Eventually, these new enjoyable reactions become automatic responses. Trauma survivors often feel that they must take everything in life very seriously, so as not to forget or diminish the trauma. They often do not feel entitled to have positive emotions.

In therapy, such reactions can be identified and addressed and, with the injection of humor, healthier reactions can be modeled, learned, and practiced. This exercise should also include having the client identify people with whom they enjoy spending time or who are supportive of them. They should be encouraged to arrange for quality time with these people and engage in fun activities with them. These activities should be logged on a calendar or a diary and reported back to the therapist. Initially, some clients may not feel entitled to engage in pleasurable activities. Incorporating fun into the therapeutic process, however, may act to lessen the feelings of survivor's guilt that may arise following a trauma in which others have suffered or perished. In some cases, it may have been years since the trauma, as with Vietnam veterans, and they have been so socially isolated in the interim that these steps require careful development and planning.

When facilitating a therapy group with survivors, getting them to focus on their humorous memories can be a means of encouraging group cohesion and validation. When they can laugh with one another and share their feelings, they can release the shame and loneliness they have attributed to their "sick" sense of humor and allow them not to feel so alone. It can be very reassuring for survivors to know that others find humor in the same things, even when they have not shared the same exact experiences. The group therapy environment also allows for individual participants to feel secure in practicing and improving their social skills with those with whom they have already established a trusting relationship.

CONCLUSION

There is rarely a satisfactory answer to questions concerning why one person has survived a traumatic event (e.g., natural disasters or combat) when others have not. Many combat veterans have such questions, however, and feel survivor's guilt when they can find no satisfactory explanation. The greater questions, therefore, involve how the survivor managed to deal with the events as they were taking place, how s/he has coped with the memories since the trauma occurred, and where the survivor's strength comes from. Among the many components that make up a person's psyche and contribute to how a situation is handled are genetic factors, upbringing, values, and prior experiences. Therapy explores all of these in order to help survivors integrate their traumatic experience(s) into who they are rather than allowing those experiences to skew that sense of identity. Determining the ways a survivor uses humor also needs to be a part of that exploration.

One's sense of humor suggests a lot about who one is and how one views the world. Understanding the ways that humor is used and its application can be very useful in the treatment of survivors. Ignoring the positive memories of a trauma survivor can cause the therapist to develop a very limited view of who that individual really is. If the therapist only looks at a survivor's negative memories, then the therapist misses part of how the individual was able to emotionally survive the trauma and how the coping skills that were used to get through the trauma can be tapped for future recovery. Using humor does not mean that the therapist needs to wear a red rubber nose during counseling sessions, although some do. Rather, it means that a survivor needs to have his/her own sense of humor validated and accepted by the therapist, particularly since humor is often integral to a sense of hope, well-being, and humanness. During the trauma, humor may have been a tool of survival; in the recovery process, it can be used as a tool for surviving and thriving as well. The role of the therapist is to help individuals (re)discover their sense of enjoyment, to use humor to alleviate stressful situations, and to confront negative thinking. As the old adage says: "Laughter is the best medicine."

REFERENCES

Adams, P. (1993). *Gesundheit!* Rochester, VT: Healing Arts Press.

Angelou, M. (1993). *Wouldn't take nothing for my journey now.* New York: Bantam Books.

Berk, L. S. (1994). New discoveries in psychoneuroimmunology. *Humor and Health Letter, 3*(6), 1-8.

Brende, J. O., & Parson, E. R. (1985). *Vietnam veterans: The road to recovery.* New York: Plenum Press.

Cousins, N. (1979). *Anatomy of an illness.* New York: Bantam Books.

Curtis, A. M. (2001, Winter). Schtick happens: The power of humor, Part II. *Trauma Lines Newsletter,* 7-8.

Doka, K. (1996). *Living with grief after sudden loss.* Washington, DC: Taylor and Francis.

Ellis, A., & Abrams, M. (1994). *How to cope with a fatal illness: The rational management of death and dying.* New York: Barricade Books, Inc.

Figley, C. R. (1995). *Compassion fatigue.* New York: Brunner/Mazel, Publishers.

Foa, E. B., Keane, T. M., & Friedman, M. J. (2000). *Effective treatments for PTSD.* New York: Guilford Press.

Friedman, M. J. (2000). *Post traumatic stress disorder: The latest assessment and treatment strategies.* Kansas City, MO: Compact Clinicals.

Fry, W. F. (2000). Humor and synergy. *Humor and Health Journal, 9*(3), 1-3.

Fry, W. F., & Salameh, W. A. (1987). *Handbook of humor and psychotherapy.* Sarasota, FL: Professional Resources Exchange, Inc.

Fry, W. F., & Salameh, W. A. (1993). *Advances in humor and psychotherapy.* Sarasota, FL: Professional Resource Press.

Lipman, S. (1991). *Laughter in hell: The use of humor during the Holocaust.* Northvale, NJ: Jason Aranson, Inc.

Marcus, N. N. (1990). Treating those who fail to take themselves seriously: Pathological aspects of humor. *American Journal of Psychotherapy, 44,* 423-332.

Tobin, D. R. (1999). *Peaceful dying.* Reading, MA: Perseus Books.

Art Speaks in Healing Survivors of War: The Use of Art Therapy in Treating Trauma Survivors

Barbara Ann Baker

SUMMARY. Mental health clinics can use creative art therapies as a means of reaching out to war refugees in their communities who may not respond to traditional talk therapy. In this case, the use of quilting and other artwork was utilized by the staff at Chicago Health Outreach to assist displaced Bosnians to cope with their war-related trauma and integration into their new environment in the United States. It can be difficult to reach refugee populations within a community whose culture and language are different from the majority, but finding other means of communicating can make a real difference for these individuals as they find safety and understanding by working on and sharing special creative projects. *[Article copies available for a fee from The Haworth Document Delivery Service: 1-800-HAWORTH. E-mail address: <docdelivery@haworthpress.com> Website: <http://www.HaworthPress.com> © 2006 by The Haworth Press, Inc. All rights reserved.]*

KEYWORDS. Creative Art Therapy, war trauma, Story Quilt, refugees, healing

Address correspondence to Barbara Ann Baker (E-mail: srgingerich@ yahoo.com).

[Haworth co-indexing entry note]: "Art Speaks in Healing Survivors of War: The Use of Art Therapy in Treating Trauma Survivors." Baker, Barbara Ann. Co-published simultaneously in *Journal of Aggression, Maltreatment & Trauma* (The Haworth Maltreatment & Trauma Press, an imprint of The Haworth Press, Inc.) Vol. 12, No. 1/2, 2006, pp. 183-198; and: *Trauma Treatment Techniques: Innovative Trends* (ed: Jacqueline Garrick, and Mary Beth Williams) The Haworth Maltreatment & Trauma Press, an imprint of The Haworth Press, Inc., 2006, pp. 183-198. Single or multiple copies of this article are available for a fee from The Haworth Document Delivery Service [1-800-HAWORTH, 9:00 a.m. - 5:00 p.m. (EST). E-mail address: docdelivery@haworthpress.com].

My artwork is my healing, my opportunity to be the real me,

To let others know that we can heal from the horrors of the past.

Thomas N. Bills, Vietnam veteran

(Handel, 1995, p. 31)

Through art expression, fractured parts of the self are brought to the surface to be observed and evaluated for change. In the process of creating visual dialogue through art, survivors of trauma are able to resolve conflict, develop personal strengths, and heal their invisible wounds. Art reaches across cultures, creating an alternate language that can be used to dissipate the effects of trauma. Artwork provides a chance to "tell secrets" without fear of retaliation. Creative art therapy is used to provide a safe atmosphere for refugees to "heal from the horrors" of war. "The emphases in art therapy for this population [trauma victims] is gathering what is unspeakable, projecting it onto the art medium and converting it into verbal testimony" (Williams & Sommer, 1994, p. 351). Art becomes a pathway to empower clients to become survivors instead of victims. The goal of the art therapist is to assist the client in achieving a healthy self and facilitate wholeness.

Chicago Health Outreach, a partner of Heartland Alliance, provides paths from harm to hope through health care, housing, and human services. The agency has accepted art therapy as a viable method of working with immigrants, refugees, and the chronically mentally ill homeless. Clients have experienced trauma and displacement either because of war, political unrest, poverty, or mental illness.

TARGET GROUPS

This article primarily focuses on the Bosnian Mental Health Program, a division of Chicago Health Outreach. The concentration is the use of art therapy with Bosnian refugees over a five-year time period. All participants in the men and women's group are over age fifty-five and came to the United States as refugees. They came from the region of Prijedor, site of the most notorious concentration camp and some of the worst destruction. The proposed goals of both groups were to increase client's social interaction with their families and the larger community, thus reducing isolation. "Being accepted by others is crucial in the healing process and the return to effective functioning in order to be hopeful of the future" (Handel, Steidle, Zacek, & Zacek, 1995, pp. 4-5). The lack of finances and language barrier results in refugees being isolated and with limited social interaction within the larger community. Activities were planned around their prewar experiences and occupations, thus rejoining them with their lost culture. The two groups met once a week for an hour and a half. The primary feature of this article will be how needlecraft and making a "Story Quilt" was used for trauma resolution.

INTERPRETER

When one cannot speak a client's language, it is necessary to work with an interpreter. Lee (1997) defines an interpreter in the following way: "A 'cultural interpreter' is an active participant in a cross-cultural/lingual interaction, assisting the provider to understand the beliefs and practices of the client's culture and assisting the client in understanding the dominant culture, by providing cultural as well as linguistic links" (p. 478). Success depends on the interpreter being the voice and bridge to the client. The interpreter for the men's group was a Bosnian physician who was separated from his family and held in a concentration camp prior to coming to the United States. Before meeting with the clients, he explained to this author the history of the region over the past 600 years and how that history evolved into the war in Bosnia. Using a map, he located and defined the different regions of Croatia, Bosnia, and Serbia before and after the war. The interpreter also gave an overview of the culture and explained the pre-refugee roles of each family member.

The circumstances of the war changed family structure within some refugee families. In rural areas, men traditionally have a higher status than women. Men work and provide for their families financially. A woman's role is to take care of the home and children. Often, as refugees, the roles are reversed, causing conflict within the family. The male head of the household may no longer be able to support his family. In some families, the wife may become more employable than the husband. Further, three generations often live together in order to combine resources. Periodically, parents have to rely on children and grandchildren for financial support. It is more common for children to learn a new language more quickly than do adults. In fact, some adults do not learn how to speak English. This is especially difficult for young children who, after a few years, stop speaking their native language and are no longer able to communicate with their parents. The language barrier often causes additional anxiety and inhibits achieving a healthy self.

It is important to be culturally sensitive to a refugee's concept of mental health. In Bosnia, as in many cultures, therapy was acceptable only for the mentally ill. Before the war, Bosnia did not have organized mental health services and counseling. Hospitals for the mentally ill and psychiatrists who gave medications did not counter the stigma of shame associated with emotional problems and mental illness. There was concern that an emotionally disturbed person would not be able to function and take care of him or her self.

Meeting with the interpreter after each session helped leaders to explore cultural issues and bring clarification for further understanding of the client's experiences. Because translating traumatic experiences can be emotionally difficult, it is important to be sensitive and respectful of the interpreter's feelings. As noted by Lee (1997), "Clinicians must encourage the interpreter to tell them when he or she is having difficulty" (p. 488).

TRAUMA

Displaced Bosnians have psychological wounds resulting from experiences of torture, massacre, ethnic cleansing, internment, rape, daily mortar and sniper fire, injury, deprivation, and loss of family and friends. For refugees, these war traumas are augmented by the stresses of living in another culture, learning the host language, finding work, dealing with new customs, schools, laws, and being alone in a foreign culture. For example, without an interpreter, clients are unable to explain their medical problems to a doctor or hospital. Thus, for example, a client's surgery was postponed because she could not communicate with the doctors. Others find asking for directions or filling out job applications difficult tasks to do independently.

Posttraumatic stress creates a variety of problems that inhibit the daily functioning of refugees. Depression, anxiety attacks, and memory loss are common. Recurrent and intrusive recollections of torture, distressing dreams, and difficulty in concentration hinder their quality of life. Bosnian women reported that they forgot how to do tasks they had done most of their life, such as baking bread and doing cultural needlework. Within the family structure, war experiences and even prewar experiences were not discussed. Seligman (1995) notes that "Social support systems are crucial at times of stress because they provide emotional support, underline the existing resources in contrast to what is lost, offer alternative ways of coping, and remind one of his or her pre-crisis identity" (p. 121). Without any emotional support, all previous identity is gone. Trust and hope for the future are often diminished.

ARTISTIC EXPRESSION

Through the art making process, a visual dialogue emerges to allow refugees to unravel fragments of their stories. Art provides a focus for self-exploration and discussion. The artwork serves as a voice for what cannot be said in words. As noted by McMurray (1988), "Artistic expression is a doorway to insight, depth communication, and healing . . . Images show us the unknown faces of our soul and generate energy for change" (p. 12). The images come forth when clients are ready to give verbal testimony. The reality of the trauma and its consequences–fear, mistrust, physical and emotional impairment–are brought to the surface. The artwork becomes an avenue to facilitate the documentation of the experience, which is validating to the survivor. Through this process, healing begins to take place.

James and Johnson (1997) state, "The creative arts therapies have firmly established themselves in the treatment regimen for Posttraumatic Stress Disorder (PTSD) patients. Because many traumatic memories are coded nonverbally in kinesthetic and visual forms, the nonverbal media of the creative art therapies are able to facilitate access to these memories" (pp. 383-384). Visual images are easier for the mind to retain than language. When traumatic events are repressed in a person's memory, good memories are also often repressed. That is, "If the torture survivor is depressed, he or she will have difficulty remembering pleasant experiences from the past" (Basoglu, 1992, p. 259). Through art, the art therapist can assist the client to uncover memories and skills of life before the trauma.

It is important to try to reconnect a person to his/her lost culture. Needlework was the collective bond of the Grandmother's group. In the beginning, the women worked independently on various needle projects. Slowly, they relearned some of the skills they had lost during their war experiences. At the same time, other skills, such as cooking and baking bread, returned. As an example, a client lived with her youngest son who was injured during the war. Before the war, she was a widow who took care of her family, a large home with a garden, and farm animals. When she migrated to the United States, she had few resources and was completely isolated. She reported, "I was so sick, mentally traumatized, that I forgot everything. I was not able to do hand work or housework." After working with peers doing needlework in group therapy, the client said that she was "very happy to be able to do things again. In the beginning I was unable to do anything." Thus, reviving pre-trauma interests led to renewed interests and creative expression. Her self-confidence emerged and this client had a new identity and purpose.

MEN'S GROUPS

The men's group was the first therapy group for Bosnian men at the agency. Having a female therapist and using art as a means of dialogue to work with men were unusual concepts for this group. In Bosnian culture, people do not talk to strangers about their problems and men usually socialize only with other men. For these reasons, they had a hard time opening up and talking about their feelings. An additional challenge for the men was to feel comfortable talking to a woman about their personal experiences. In the beginning, there was some resistance to making art because a common perception is that "art is for children" and men are supposed to be involved in serious things. In other words, art was considered play. In rural Bosnia, a man who made art, music, or who danced as a job was considered weak. Art could be considered only as a hobby. With the support of the interpreter and patience, the men began to open up and trust enough to do artwork and talk about their lives and trauma. Drawing, painting, and sculpture materials were used. This artwork was a catalyst to promote discussion.

To assist the clients to feel more comfortable, the therapist developed exercises around first memories of their childhood. These exercises revealed that all of the clients had experienced the trauma of World War II, and some had lost parents in that war. As children, they had learned about the devastation of war and poverty. As adults, they re-experienced some of the same events. This time they were the widows and parents who lost their homes and their country, who suffered the loss and injury of their children, and who were powerless to protect their families. For example, one client's son was taken from his home by his neighbor, never to be seen or heard from again.

When this author started working with the men's group, she found it challenging to work with an interpreter. In order to make the clients feel more comfortable, this author would have the clients do artwork and write about their feelings and experiences, then the interpreter would translate their writing. One client began writing every day. As a child, he was denied a formal education because men in the rural areas were destined to be laborers. When he was sixteen, he pursued and received an education. This warranted him several promotions in his job as a fireman in a paper factory, which he held for thirty years before retiring. During his free time, he worked as a stonecutter and made monuments. He also built his own as well as his son's home. Prior to art therapy, this client did no formal writing. Five years later, he is still writing and hopes someday to have his writings published. He said,

> It's not comfortable meeting someone for the first time. It's not easy to talk about things that happened. When you use a pen and start drawing, you don't think about how to talk. . . . Through the artwork, it helped to calm me down because I got through horrible things and my nerves were not so good. It worked for me. The writing helped me to concentrate. . . . I found myself in my writing. I didn't think about anything else. I go to my room and write. . . . When I am finished, I feel different. I feel satisfied. After our sessions, I would put it on my paper my way. . . . No one in Bosnia (rural) wrote a book. I think it is important for people to know what happened so it does not happen again.

This client wants to tell his story so future generations will know what happened in Bosnia. In one session, he drew a picture of twelve men with ropes around their necks and said, "I saw these twelve men being hung. I have not been able to talk about it till now." The drawing helped him tell what happened, and his artwork and writing have given him new purpose and hope for the future.

Several months after the group began, a fifty-eight-year-old client joined the group. Prior to attending, he was so traumatized that he had to be hospitalized. The client had little social contact and was very isolated because he found being with other people difficult. In the beginning, he initially resisted making art. With encouragement, he slowly began to respond to art therapy and socialize with the other men. At first, he was able to tolerate coming only every other week. After two months, he started coming every week. Each week, there was a noticeable improvement in his participation and socialization. The content of his drawings changed from just a few marks on paper with a pencil to very detailed colorful pictures. In one session, he drew a very vivid picture of the Mostar Bridge, an important historical landmark that was destroyed during the war. Several months later his disability benefits, which he applied for after his discharge from the hospital, were approved. However, the client decided he would rather work and got a job. He reported, "I've never felt better in my life. Thank you, I have my life back." This client was able to dissipate some of his trauma and become a productive part of the community.

The men's group lasted for six months. Each week, the art project was followed by discussion of the work and any issues that surfaced. Clients used the art process to talk about their experiences and reduce stress. Their work consisted of simple marks on paper to elaborate drawings of their homeland. Their collages portrayed their interests, such as hunting, fishing, homes, flowers, and Bosnia. One client made a clay footprint, saying that his footprint was on a beach in Bosnia and Chicago. This statement led to an interesting discussion about the client's connection to two countries. To have a record of their work, they kept it in a journal. One participant took his journal home and returned the next week with the journal filled with newspaper clippings from Bosnia and pictures from magazines. Through his journal images, he was able to tell stories about what happened in Bosnia and life before the war. The men used the art to talk about painful and joyful experiences of their childhood, their homes, work, family, and their trauma. Through this process, the men got their dignity back and moved forward with their lives. Because of the success of this group, an art therapy men's group was formed. One man decided to join this second group.

The second group consisted of four men with various backgrounds. Two of the men were friends prior to attending the sessions. The men in the second group were more traumatized and had concurrent physical and mental impairments. Each client was asked to give his name, address, and list his problems. One client had lost his daughter and two other members of his family in a car accident three months prior to joining the group. This client talked about the accident only once, in an individual session two years after the accident. Another client said, "Sometimes I do not know my name or my address. I have experienced so much trauma that I sometimes get lost outside my building and can't find my way home."

The next week, the same client brought in a video about his son and the war in Bosnia. There was concern that this would be too difficult for the men to see. However, the men insisted that they see the video. Viewed during two sessions, time was allowed to discuss and process the disturbing images. During this therapist's training, an art therapy professor cautioned, "Try not to let clients leave in an emotionally vulnerable state." This helpful advice meant that, at the end of each session, time was allowed for discussion, composure, and a refocus to the present. Even though it was a very abrupt beginning, it established a credibility that this author was willing to see and hear about the horror of the client's trauma experiences.

Flexibility was the key to the success of this group. The challenge was to come up with creative ways to introduce the art materials. When things got too intense, each person was given a brush and one color of paint. A very large piece of paper covered two tables. The directions were to paint, keep moving around the paper, and not to put too much focus on subject matter and composition while painting. Just have fun and listen to the music of Paul Simon's "Graceland" while painting. "Graceland" was chosen because of its upbeat rhythm. This activity resulted in a very meaningful mural. One of the men painted the word Bosnia. Since there was no one direction, when asked which way the mural should be displayed, they responded by saying Bosnia should be upside down, referring to how "everything in Bosnia is turned upside down, nothing is the same as it was before the war." Afterwards, they processed the experience and images. Other times, various materials were put on the table with no directive. The clients had the choice to make art or just to talk. Eventually, the client who resisted making art the most started making art.

One of the most important aspects of the group was to provide a safe place for the men to talk about their experiences. They had questions about everything, including politics, human behavior, American culture, etc. Art was often used to illustrate and facilitate further discussion. It was easier for the men to tell their stories, ask questions, and understand with the use of visuals. During the art therapy process, clients became less anxious, their somatic symptoms lessened, and the quality of their lives improved.

GRANDMOTHER'S GROUP

The creative art of needlecraft is practiced throughout the world. In Bosnia, needlecraft is an important aspect of culture for women. It gives them a sense of identity and serves as a way to express their individualism. The use of needlecraft with clients lowered their stress, reduced tension, increased concentration, and promoted self-exploration and healing. The Grandmother's Group worked with various methods of needlecraft as a common interest to facilitate the women in coming together and socializing. The group projects consisted of embroidery, needlepoint, crochet, knitting, needle-lace, and quilting. A Story Quilt project provided the women with the means to honor memories of loved ones, a lost country, and culture so they were not forgotten.

The women in this group were some of the first Bosnian refugees to come to the agency. In the beginning, they had physical and mental impairment, loss of memory, disorganization, and were isolated with little social support. All of the women had done various forms of needlecraft before the war. However, because of their trauma, they had impaired abilities. The focus was to have them meet each week at the agency to socialize and reduce isolation while a psychology intern and an art therapy intern, who had no previous experience working with needlecraft, facilitated. The women brought in coffee and cultural food, and eventually began to trust each other and the facilitators. The women agreed that they wanted to do needlework. To assist in dialoguing and understanding, the interns brought in books and magazines for ideas. The women decided to do individual projects at home and then during session put them together into one banner. Over a period of three months, they assembled eight panels plus borders with Bosnian symbols, flowers, and scenes. Through this process, the women's memory improved and their daily functioning increased, they became less anxious and less isolated, and they formed friendships within the group. The banner project gave the women a renewed purpose to their lives. This author facilitated the group when the interns completed their internship.

The women's social skills slowly returned and outside activities in their homes improved. Gradually, some of their memory returned, but they did not reveal the details of their personal traumas. Instead, they talked about news from Bosnia, family, and neighbors. The interpreter, a young Bosnian female, said they did not want to talk about unpleasant things. Slowly, they began to trust each other and the content and quality of their needlework increased. Several of the women did very elaborate needlepoint and embroidery pictures depicting life in Bosnia as well as needle-lace, needlepoint, crocheting, and knitting.

One client came every week but was very quiet during sessions and did not work on a project. After five weeks, she was asked if there was anything this author could buy her to work with. She said, "Wool." At that time, we had some thread for crochet, and embroidery materials, but there was no yarn. After buying her yarn, she began to participate. Prior to coming to the United States, she could not read or write. As she slowly began to increase her self-confidence, she eventually learned to read and write in English. She embroidered a large banner honoring Kosorac, her village of twenty-five thousand people that had been destroyed during the war. This memorial, depicting the Bosnian flag, gave the client a safe way to talk about the destruction of her village.

The women slowly began to talk about their personal traumas. Initially, they talked superficially about losing their husbands, family members, and homes. However, they did not go into detail about their experiences. After a year and a half, one client talked about her nineteen-year-old son who was missing since the early part of the war. A news report said that one of the mass graves near her village was being opened and she was anxious that they would find her son. Eventually, the women began to talk about more personal experiences, mostly centered on events in the news or reports and pictures from family members who had returned from trips to Bosnia. At this time, they were still doing individual projects. Through an individual session with a client, this author discovered that the client's mother made quilts. None of the women had ever done any form of quilting before.

STORY QUILTS

Needlecraft and quilting is part of this author's heritage passed down from one generation to the next. Just as in this author's grandmother's and mother's generations, women from all over the world have come together to share their joys and sorrows and to diminish isolation. Often in rural areas, isolated from the outside world and some houses without electricity, they would meet in each other's homes or the area churches. They would share news, talk about their difficulties, families, neighbors, and gossip. This was their means of healing from loneliness, the hardship of domestic life, and to get through traumatic events. The craft of quilting and the "Quilting Bee" became a therapeutic tool for healing to take place.

"Story Panels" are a venue for cultures to pass stories of their history to future generations. For example, the 231-foot-long Bayeux Tapestry, which is over 1,000 years old, depicts the Norman conquest of England in 1066, while a 272-foot long, 3 foot high panel made of bits of cloth needlework commemorates the 1944 "Operation Overlord, D-Day and the Battle of Normandy." Both panels tell the story as significant historical documents. Charles de Gaulle said, " Weapons have both tortured and shaped the world. Shameful and magnificent, their story is the story of man" (as cited in Foote, 1994, p. 80). Happily, that story can sometimes be recorded with a needle.

African art and folk art history emphasize the importance of quilt making. "Quilt patterns and stitches were used in the struggle for freedom–as codes that could be read by enslaved blacks as they traveled along the Underground Railroad. . . . Decorative arts–particularly quilts–go far beyond their functional nature . . . the beauty, the grace, the mastery, the spirituality, the sensuality and the communicative power of quilts. . . . There is a connection between the quilts as an instrument of freedom in the nineteenth century and as a didactic medium for the story quilts of today" (Tobin & Dobard, 1999, p. xx). The West African kingdom of the Dahomey tells their history through wall hangings. Each symbol or animal is carefully appliquéd onto cloth to represent a king or event from the past. In Liberia, only "happy women" are allowed to work the cloth. Dendel (1974) notes that, "African craftsmen seem to have an instinct for 'what the cloth says'. . . tiny scraps can be made to 'talk.' What these scraps say in appliqués of the Dahomey is the history of a people" (p. 16). Many folk artists often make art from materials found in their environment to assist them in recovery from difficulties and traumas in their lives. In Mexico, Central and South American countries, people make fabric "story panels" to tell about their lives. Symbols and pictures are used to explore the events in their lives.

Making a group story quilt was a process for the Bosnian women to reconnect with an aspect of their culture and gave them a way to tell their stories. The "story quilt" was a visual record of survivors' lives. Through books, magazines, and quilt shows, the group researched how to tell their stories through a story quilt. The women drew pictures of their homes before the war. Ellen Anne Eddy, a famous quilt maker, loaned her quilt books and solicited materials from fellow quilt makers. Ms. Eddy and her friend, Ms. Mary, came to a session to demonstrate how to construct a story quilt. They put together a sample quilt depicting and memorializing a client's son missing since the beginning of the war. The women brought Bosnian food and coffee to show their appreciation. This event was a great success and helped to dissipate some of the women's fear of working with an unfamiliar craft and materials. Although they were very skilled in various forms of needlework, they had to be taught how to join tiny pieces of materials together and how to appliqué.

Next, they reviewed their drawings, materials were selected, and technique demonstrated. After a few weeks, they were ready to take the materials home and work on their individual panels. The women brought in five story panels, varying in size, character, and rendering, that depicted aspects of the interior or exteriors of their homes, yards, farms, and Bosnia. One woman made a quilt square similar to the style of quilt that her mother had made. As they proceeded, the women began to reveal more about their personal lives before the war and slowly began to talk about their trauma experiences.

Although the panels were very unique, the project needed something to make it into a completed quilt. Group members looked through quilt books to decide what should be added. The decision was made to add female figures with long dresses as self-portraits, as well as appliqués of their houses. Their drawings served as templates for patterns and fabric selection. Two weeks later, the women brought in the work that became a turning point for the project. Instead of self-portrait figures and houses to appliqué onto the quilt, they brought in new story panels. The women began to tell specific details about their lives and their traumas through the additional panels. One client said that, in her village, the color white was considered a symbol for royalty. However, they were being forced to put white in the windows to signify that they were Muslims. The client said that she wanted to resist, but her son said that they might be killed if they did. The client stitched white onto the windows of the house in her panel. Another client made a panel with several houses, mountains, and hills to depict her village. Her female figure was a refugee with a sack to hold her only possessions. A white band was stitched onto one of the arms of the figure. She said that in the concentration and refugee camp, she and others had to wear white bands around their arms to indicate that they were different and Muslims.

It is important to note that after the quilt project started, we got a new interpreter, a Bosnian physician. The maturity of the interpreter helped the women to feel more at ease in telling their stories. She explained the significance of putting white in the window and wearing white armbands. It was mandatory and a person risked being killed if they did not comply. This information led to a discussion of the similarity to the Holocaust, except the armbands were yellow and symbolized being Jewish.

Some panels also had references to World War II. One client said that the female figure in her second panel was of "a bad woman who did many terrible things. My husband and cousin were her first victims. The bad woman's father did terrible things during World War II. The bad woman was worse than the father." This same client said that "The family dog," in her original panel, "was a very brave dog, warning the family saved them from being killed." The enemy cut off the dog's legs for revenge.

One of the women had not brought in a panel. She said that her family threw away her panel of a vase of flowers. She carefully selected fabrics and asked to take them home. The next week, she came in with a very large panel. The panel had various materials glued to the surface that represented a footprint, a river, skulls, flowers, animals, etc. She told us about the myth of Kozaroc and Mohammed's mother, Fatima, and how she turned the sea into a river, leaving her footprint on the mountain 3,900 years ago. This place was considered a "sacred and happy place" and many people went there to hide from the enemy. The client reported that 1,600 people were killed at this location. When this author asked her who was the figure in her panel, she responded, "It is a mother who is trying to find her children and she is crying." The quilt became a memorial to their past and the trauma they experienced. It was their way to tell their stories.

The same client reported that making the quilt made her "very sad. I saw everything what I experienced before. It was heartbreaking what I experienced there. I have seen everything, when they hit and beat children, when they raped and took the children. I do not know where. It was not easy working on the quilt and it took almost a year. During this work, we were all the time thinking. Afterwards, when we don't remember everything, it was better. It helped us to feel better. It's not so easy to be alone. It is better to be together. When I am working with my hands, I don't remember what happened to me. The work helps you forget."

The original resistance we encountered to working in an unfamiliar medium dissipated. This is demonstrated by one client who said, "The quilt–small pieces of fabric–I imagined to be horrible not able to do anything when finished. When I saw work of peers, I was so excited and amazed. It helped us a lot to work in a group." The women supported each other and, as they worked together on the quilt, developed friendships within the group and became very close.

CONCLUSION

Randall and Lutz (1991) note, "Survivors who have difficulty grieving or expressing their feelings about loved ones who have been killed or who 'disappeared' may be helped by creating actual or symbolic memorials. These memorials serve as a concrete symbol through which previously inaccessible feelings about the loss of these loved ones can be expressed and worked through" (p. 123). The memorials produced by the Bosnians serve to honor the memories of their loved ones, their lost country, and their culture so they are not forgotten. Memorials are very important in the healing process and serve as a means of dialogue to the community. The Bosnian Women's Quilt is made with love and tears for that which was lost. It tells their stories to a larger community so people will know what happened to them. As one client said to a group of friends and counselors at the agency, "In the beginning we resisted working on the project. However, we are so glad that we continued. It was hard to remember all that happened to us. The quilt has given us back part of our soul."

Wadeson, Dirkin, and Perach (1989) stated, "Only silence is enough to contain the horror" (p. 7). Through the art-making process, trauma survivors are able to create visual dialogue to tell the "horrors" of their experiences so healing may take place. As noted by Basoglu (1992), "The voice of the torture survivor is a whisper. Where this voice can be heard is in the literature of survivors, i.e., in their art, poems, stories and biographies—and not in the medical literature" (p. 25). Art is an avenue to empowerment and wholeness. "Art, more than almost any other human activity, can nurture and enhance life: the life of the human spirit, the life of the imagination, and physical life itself. . . . Art, above all else, allows us mere mortals a glimpse, if only momentarily, of eternal truths" (Kinkade, 2002, p. 16).

REFERENCES

Basoglu, M. (1992). *Torture and its consequences*. New York: Cambridge University Press.

Dendel, E. W. (1974). *African fabric crafts*. Marlboro, NJ: Taplinger Publishing Co.

Foote, T. (1994, May). Tapestried tales of the two rough Channel Crossings. *Smithsonian, 25*(2), 68-81.

Handel, S., Steidle, A., Zacek, G., & Zacek, R. (1995). *Soldiers heart: Survivor's view of combat trauma*. Lutherville, MD: Sidran.

James, M., & Johnson, D. R. (1997). Drama therapy in the treatment of combat-related post-traumatic stress disorder. *The Arts in Psychotherapy, 23*(5), 383-395.

Kinkade,T. (2002, April). Sharing the light. *American Artist*, p. 16.

Lee, E. (1997). Cross-cultural communication: Therapeutic use of interpreters. In E. Lee (Ed.), *Working with Asian Americans* (pp. 477-489). New York: Guilford Press

McMurray, M. (1988). *Illuminations: The healing image*. Berkeley: Winglow.

Randall, G. R., & Lutz, E. L. (1991). *Serving survivors of torture*. Washington, DC: AAAS.

Seligman, Z. (1995). Trauma and drama: A lesson from the concentration camps. *The Arts in Psychotherapy, 22*(2), 119-132.

Tobin, J. L., & Dobard, R. (1999). *In plain view. The secret story of quilts and the underground railroad.* New York: Random House

Wadeson, H., Dirkin, J., & Perach, D. (1989). *Advances in art therapy.* New York: Wiley & Sons.

Williams, M. B., & Sommer, J. F. (1994). *Handbook of post-traumatic therapy.* Westport, CT: Greenwood.

Virtual Reality Exposure for Veterans with Posttraumatic Stress Disorder

David J. Ready
Stacey Pollack
Barbara Olasov Rothbaum
Renato D. Alarcon

SUMMARY. Two open trials of Virtual Reality based exposure therapy (VRE) to desensitize Vietnam veterans with Posttraumatic Stress Disorder (PTSD) to some of their traumatic memories are described. A total of 21 patients were exposed to one of two virtual Vietnam computer-generated environments in which their individual traumatic experiences were simulated in response to their recounting these events. Although two patients experienced significant increases in symptoms during VRE, all patients' PTSD symptoms were below baseline by the 3-month post-treatment assessment. When the data from the two open trials was combined, clinically meaningful and statistically significant reductions in PTSD symptoms were found. These changes were long lasting as evidenced by the 6-month follow-up assessments. Two case examples are provided and future applications of this treatment are discussed. *[Article copies available for a fee from The Haworth Document Delivery Service: 1-800-HAWORTH. E-mail address: <docdelivery@haworthpress.com> Website: <http://www.HaworthPress.com> © 2006 by The Haworth Press, Inc. All rights reserved.]*

Address correspondence to David J. Ready, Atlanta VA Medical Center (116A-4), 1670 Clarimont Road, Decatur, GA (E-mail: David.Ready@med.va.gov).

The authors would like to acknowledge the invaluable contribution of Dr. Larry Hodges, Ken Graap, Greg Inman, Fran Shahar, and Dr. David Baltzell to this project.

[Haworth co-indexing entry note]: "Virtual Reality Exposure for Veterans with Posttraumatic Stress Disorder." Ready, David J. et al. Co-published simultaneously in *Journal of Aggression, Maltreatment & Trauma* (The Haworth Maltreatment & Trauma Press, an imprint of The Haworth Press, Inc.) Vol. 12, No. 1/2, 2006, pp. 199-220; and: *Trauma Treatment Techniques: Innovative Trends* (ed: Jacqueline Garrick, and Mary Beth Williams) The Haworth Maltreatment & Trauma Press, an imprint of The Haworth Press, Inc., 2006, pp. 199-220. Single or multiple copies of this article are available for a fee from The Haworth Document Delivery Service [1-800-HAWORTH, 9:00 a.m. - 5:00 p.m. (EST). E-mail address: docdelivery@haworthpress.com].

KEYWORDS. Virtual Reality therapy, PTSD, Exposure therapy, Vietnam veterans

INTRODUCTION

According to the American Psychiatric Association's *Diagnostic and Statistical Manual* (DSM-IV; 1994), Posttraumatic Stress Disorder (PTSD) is an anxiety disorder characterized by the re-experiencing of traumatic events, emotional numbing and avoidance, and increased arousal. PTSD is the most common and disabling psychopathological condition affecting the veteran population. A 1992 study estimated that 830,000 Vietnam veterans suffered from chronic combat related PTSD (Weiss et al., 1992). Over 180,000 veterans have sought treatment from the Department of Veterans Affairs (VA) Medical Centers for PTSD, and the VA has classified over 153,000 veterans as disabled by PTSD (Rosenheck, Spencer, & Gray, 2002). In response, the Department of Veterans Affairs has set up 145 specialized PTSD treatment programs in VA Medical Centers and 206 Vet Centers that also serve a large number of PTSD veterans. Unfortunately, outcome studies of VA PTSD treatment have been disappointing (Zadecki, 1999). Although some studies of VA PTSD treatment have reported positive results, these studies often do not include post-treatment follow-up assessments (e.g., Frueh, Turner, Beidel, Mirabella, & Jones, 1996). This is a critical omission given that studies of VA PTSD programs that included follow-up assessment found, in almost every case, a rebound to pretreatment symptom levels when the follow-up assessments occurred at or after six months (Hammarberg & Silver, 1994; Zadecki, 1999).

Additional studies report positive outcomes but there are questions about the clinical significance of the findings (Hammarberg & Silver, 1994). For example, a study of 554 patients being treated in six different VA outpatient PTSD Clinical Teams reported significant reductions in PTSD symptoms on the Mississippi Scale after four months of treatment (Fontana, Rosenheck, & Spencer, 1993). However, there was only a mean change from 122.67 at admission to 121.24 at four months on the Mississippi Scale. This change is far less than one standard deviation, which is 18, and still well above the usual cutoff for a PTSD diagnosis, which is 107 (Keane, Caddell, & Taylor, 1988). That is, although these changes were statistically significant, they may not be clinically significant. Of even greater concern is a study that found veterans had significantly more PTSD symptoms following an intensive inpatient VA treatment program (Johnson, Rosenheck, Fontana, Lubin, Charney, & Southwick, 1996).

There is evidence that veterans, particularly Vietnam veterans, are more difficult to treat than other PTSD patient populations, as is noted in the recently published, empirically based treatment guidelines for PTSD (Foa, Keane, & Friedman, 2000). To date there is very little empirical evidence that contemporary therapies produce clinically significant and enduring reductions in PTSD symptoms with American combat veterans (Zadecki, 1999).

Exposure-Based Treatments for PTSD

There is more empirical support for the efficacy of exposure therapy than for any other form of treatment for PTSD (Rothbaum, Meadows, Resick, & Foy, 2000). Exposure treatments for PTSD generally involve repeated imaginal reliving of the trauma with the aim of facilitating its processing, a mechanism presumably impaired in individuals with chronic PTSD (Foa, Steketee, & Rothbaum, 1989). The efficacy of Imaginal Exposure (IE) for treating PTSD has been demonstrated in several case reports of US war veterans (Fairbank, Gross, & Keane, 1983; Johnson, Gilmore, & Shenoy, 1982; Keane & Kaloupek, 1982).

Only five controlled studies have examined the usefulness of IE in the treatment of VA patients with PTSD (Boudewyns, Hyer, Woods, Harrison, & McCrame, 1990; Cooper & Clum, 1989; Glynn et al., 1999; Keane, Fairbank, Caddell, & Zimmering, 1989; Schnurr et al., 2003). Four found that participants experienced some benefit from receiving IE treatment compared to control subjects, but the effects were often small (Rothbaum, Hodges, Ready, Graap, & Alarcon, 2001). Two of these studies found that IE produced clinically significant and lasting (at six month follow-up) reductions in the positive symptoms of PTSD (i.e., re-experiencing and hyperarousal), but did not significantly reduce the avoidance and numbing symptoms (Cooper & Clum, 1989; Glynn et al., 1999).

A recent multi-site study used a novel group approach to IE, but did not find IE to be more effective than a control condition (Schnurr et al., 2003). In this study, participants were only asked to recount their traumatic experiences during group therapy a total of two or three times. (Generally, when IE is used in individual psychotherapy, patients are asked to describe their trauma eight or more times; Foa & Rothbaum, 1998.) One possible explanation for this study's failure to find support for IE is that it did not require an adequate amount of exposure.

There has been some support for the utility of Eye Movement Desensitization and Reprocessing therapy (EMDR), a type of cognitive behavioral therapy with a strong exposure component with veterans (Lipke & Botkin, 1992; Shapiro, 1999). However, studies of EMDR with combat veterans that include six-month or longer post-treatment assessments showed a symptom-rebound effect similar to that described above (Devilly, Spence, & Rapee, 1998; Macklin, Metzger, Lasko, Berry, Orr, & Pittman, 2000).

Although it is generally agreed that exposure therapy is the most effective treatment for PTSD, it has been greatly underutilized with veterans (Boudewyns, 1994). This underutilization may be due to the difficulty of doing imaginal exposure with combat veterans and the impracticality of providing in vivo combat exposure. Many Vietnam veterans find it very difficult to stick with their traumatic memories long enough to allow habituation through imaginal exposure (Boudewyns, 1994). We believe that one possible explanation for this difficulty is the habit strength built up by their partially successful attempts to avoid these same memories for over thirty years.

VIRTUAL REALITY

Virtual Reality (VR) utilizes technology that integrates real-time computer graphics, body-tracking devices, visual displays, and other sensory input devices. Patients wear a head-mounted display (HMD) fitted with an electromagnetic sensor and stereo headphones. As an individual looks forward in an HMD, s/he is presented with a stereoscopic computer-generated view of a virtual world that changes in a natural way as his/her head and body move. When the patient wears the HMD, computer screens take up the patient's entire visual field, and the audio effects controlled by the therapist dominate his/her hearing. What distinguishes VR from seeing a video or an interactive computer game is the sense of being immersed in and present within the computer-generated environment.

With the availability of VR technology, a new form of exposure therapy has developed. Virtual Reality Exposure (VRE) therapy appears to have several advantages over the traditional treatment protocol, including: (a) increased convenience for both the therapist and patient; (b) increased control over the exposure experience; and (c) a more engaging environment than that which can be obtained with imaginal exposures alone. Given these advantages, VRE has begun to be used in the treatment of disorders that have been successfully treated with traditional exposure therapies in the past. For example, VRE has been found to be a very useful tool in the treatment of phobias (Anderson, Rothbaum, & Hodges, 2001).

Rationale of VRE for PTSD in Veterans

Exposure therapy is a commonly used treatment for PTSD. Traditionally, exposure therapy has been difficult to apply to the treatment of Vietnam veterans with war-related PTSD for two primary reasons. First, this population has been found to be very resistant to engaging in traumatic memories of their war experiences, making imaginal exposure therapy difficult. Second, practical constraints prevent the patient from being able to repeatedly face the original feared environment (i.e., combat). VRE is a step forward in the treatment of this population, because it provides patients with a simulation of the feared environment that is realistic enough to keep them engaged in the traumatic memories and because this can be done in the convenience of the therapist's office.

VRE for PTSD was first developed to help Vietnam veterans become desensitized to some of their traumatic memories while immersed in a computer-generated "Virtual Vietnam" (Rothbaum et al., 1999). The goal of VRE is to aid individuals in emotionally processing their most traumatic Vietnam memories. This is accomplished by providing, in a graduated manner, trauma-related stimulation to assist the patient in the repeated accessing and recounting of these memories. In VRE, it is important that the patient become engaged enough with the traumatic memories without becoming emotionally overwhelmed by these memories. The patient is instructed to mentally "keep one foot in the therapist's office and the other in Vietnam." If the individual is not sufficiently engaged in the traumatic experience, he is unlikely to become desensitized to it. If the patient is too fully engaged in the traumatic experience, it is also unlikely that desensitization will occur (Rothbaum et al., 2001).

Although VR creates an artificial world, it is our observation that veterans suffering from combat-related PTSD have responded to the Virtual Vietnam environments with a strong sense of feeling present in a Vietnam-like setting. These environments contain many of the stimuli present during the veterans' traumatic experiences. Patients are exposed to these cues in such a manner as to induce partial reliving of the experience. When successful, this partial reliving facilitates the emotional processing of these traumatic memories, causing these memories to become desensitized. Desensitization of traumatic memories has been found to result in reductions of PTSD symptoms (Rothbaum et al., 1999). The goal of exposure therapy with PTSD is the same as the goal of exposure therapy with phobias: to help the individual expose her/himself to that which s/he fears in such a manner as to facilitate desensitization of the feared stimuli and, in the case of PTSD, the traumatic memories evoked by the stimuli (Rothbaum et al., 1999). Desensitization generally occurs when the individual is repeatedly exposed to that which is feared, in a manner that prevents or minimizes avoidance and eventually leads to a sense of mastery over responses to that stimulus. As with exposure therapy for phobias, exposure therapy for PTSD is conducted in a supportive environment where the connection to the therapist can help individuals tolerate the exposure to the feared stimuli. As with phobias, the intensity of exposure is increased over sessions as the individual habituates. With VRE, the therapist can control the amount of external stimuli that relates to a traumatic experience on a moment-to-moment basis while carefully monitoring the individual's responses. If the therapist can provide the appropriate level of external stimuli and help the patient not feel overwhelmed by his/her own internal stimuli, emotional processing occurs (Rothbaum et al., 1999).

METHOD

Participants

Participants were recruited through referrals from within the VA system and through local advertisements. Potential participants were screened by telephone or in person to determine eligibility for the study. Participants needed to be male Vietnam veterans in treatment for PTSD who were (a) experiencing significant symptoms of PTSD related to Vietnam combat experiences (as measured by the Clinician Administered PTSD Scale; Blake et al., 1990); and (b) either not on psychotropic medication or have been stable on such medication for at least three months. Patients with a history of a substance use disorder had to have had at least three months of sobriety. Excluded from the study were those who had a history or evidence of mania, schizophrenia, organic mental disorders or psychoses; those who had the presence of prominent suicidal ideation; and those who had histories of significant cardiac problems, seizures, or other physical limitations that would contraindicate the stress of exposure therapy. In addition, patients were excluded if the VRE stimuli that was available was inconsistent with subject's trauma (e.g., trauma from a plane crash). Finally, individuals whose primary reaction to his/her Vietnam memories is guilt rather than fear or anxiety (guilt has been shown not to be amenable to exposure techniques) were also excluded (Rothbaum et al., 2001). Following the screening, eligible participants were scheduled for an assessment with an evaluator. This assessment included obtaining informed consent, an extensive clinical interview, and the administration of the battery outlined below. The results of a combined sample of 14 patients who completed at least one post-treatment assessment in two open trials of VRE are reported here.

The single most challenging aspect of our research with VRE has been patient recruitment. Some VA staff were reluctant to refer patients to VRE due to concern that this unproven treatment would cause patients harm. Many veterans were reluctant to volunteer for the study due to suspiciousness about government studies, fear that the treatment would make them worse or a reluctance to be one of the first in the world to try a new treatment for which the outcome was unknown. Although well over one hundred patients were screened by phone and/or in person, in three years only 21 veterans were judged to be appropriate for VRE based on our inclusion and exclusion criteria and were willing to commit to treatment. Six of these dropped out during treatment. Two dropped out after their first exposure to a Virtual Vietnam environment because they feared VR would increase their symptoms, while the other four dropped out after five sessions due to their feeling that VRE was not helping them. Appropriate referrals were made for these patients, and none reported any lasting harmful effects of VRE treatment. One positive note is the fact that the dropout rate decreased significantly after the first year; in addition, the final nine patients who were recruited into the study completed the treatment.

Measures

Screening battery and outcome measures included the Clinician Administered PTSD Scale (CAPS; Blake et al., 1990). This is a 30-item interview based on the diagnostic criteria for PTSD found in the DSM IV (APA, 1994). It assesses the frequency and intensity of specific PTSD symptoms and associated features. The CAPS has been found to have excellent psychometric properties (Weathers & Litz, 1996). There is also evidence that it is sensitive to symptom change as a result of treatment (van der Kolk et al., 1994).

Self-report measures included the Impact of Events Scale (IES; Horowitz, Wilner, & Alvarez, 1979). This 15-item scale measures the intrusion and avoidance symptoms related to a specific traumatic event. Split-half reliability for total scale is .86; Cronbach's alpha was .80 for the avoidance scale, and .78 for the intrusion scale. One-week test-retest reliability was .87.

The Beck Depression Inventory (BDI; Beck, Ward, Mendelsohn, Mock, & Erbaugh, 1961) is a 21-item questionnaire that assesses numerous symptoms of depression. The authors report excellent split-half reliability (.93), and correlations with clinician ratings of depression ranging between .62 and .66.

The Subjective Units of Discomfort Scale (SUDS; Kaplan, Smith, & Coons, 1995) is a self-report measure assessing the intensity of a patient's emotional distress. Patients rate their discomfort at a given time on a scale of 0-100, with 0 representing no discomfort and 100 representing extreme discomfort.

Procedures: The VRE PTSD Treatment

In a joint project between the Atlanta VA Medical Center, Emory University, and the Georgia Institute of Technology, Vietnam veterans suffering from war-related PTSD were provided with Virtual Reality Exposure (VRE) therapy beginning in December 1997. Dr. Barbara Rothbaum was the Principal Investigator for the first open trial of VRE for PTSD, in which 16 patients started VRE, six dropped out, and one did not attend any post-treatment assessments. The Principal Investigator for a second open trial using the same methods was Dr. David Ready. Five patients completed VRE treatment with no dropouts. Dr. Ready was the primary therapist in both trials. Although the results of the first trial have already been reported (Rothbaum et al., 2001), we believe that combining all the data from both open trials presents a clearer picture of the efficacy of this new form of exposure therapy for PTSD than either one can independently.

In the two open trials, patients received two 90-minute individual therapy sessions per week on an outpatient basis. On some occasions, treatment occurred less often due to scheduling conflicts by either the patients or the therapist. The total number of sessions a patient received ranged from 8 to 20 and was determined by standardized criteria set forth in the treatment manual used by the two VRE therapists. Both VRE therapists were PhD-level Clinical Psychologists.

Two "Virtual Vietnam" environments were used. The environment that more closely resembled the patient's trauma was used with each participant. One environment resembled a Huey helicopter ride that includes several types of Vietnam-like terrain, and a scenario that resembled touching down in a "hot" landing zone. The second virtual environment was of a clearing with trees, several rolling hills, a swampy area, and a surrounding jungle that resembled a landing zone that appears about two acres wide. The patient was able to move around in this environment at will through the manipulation of a joystick.

Visual effects for the helicopter ride environment include taking off, flying over rice paddies, flying low over a river, flying near mountains, flying over thick jungle, flying up into clouds, and landing in a landing zone similar to the one described above. Audio effects include outgoing machine-gun fire, radio chatter, incoming gunfire, explosions, and yelling upon landing.

Visual effects for the landing zone environment included muzzle flashes from the jungle, a bright flash with the sound of a land mine exploding, helicopters flying overhead, helicopters landing and taking off, helicopter blades starting and stopping to rotate, darkness, and fog. The available audio effects for this environment included jungle sounds such as crickets, distant gunfire and explosions, enemy machine-gun fire, helicopters, mortars being launched and landing, rocket explosions, land mines going off, sloshing sounds in the swampy area, screaming, and male voices yelling "Move out! Move out!" The therapist had control of the intensity (volume) and duration of the sound effects. The therapist turned on or off each of the audio and visual stimuli as needed. It is important to note that the VRE environments did not have to include all elements of a traumatic experience in order to be effective. The environment did, however, have to simulate enough of the original trauma stimuli to trigger the "fear structure" (Foa & Kozak, 1986) of the patient's particular combat trauma.

Course of treatment. All veterans who expressed an interest in VRE between the dates of September 1997 and March 2001 were carefully screened as outlined above. In addition to meeting the inclusion criteria and not being ruled out by the exclusion criteria, individuals had to commit to treatment, be judged as being able to tolerate an initial increase in symptoms, and seem likely to benefit from VRE treatment.

Treatment schedule. Session one began by orienting participants to the treatment process. The therapist made sure that each participant understood the treatment rationale and the possible risks and benefits of participating in VRE, and answered participants' questions. Participants were told that the treatment may initially intensify their symptoms and cause them to think about Vietnam more frequently, but that, while unpleasant, both experiences usually signified that therapy was successfully helping them to confront and process previously avoided material. It was critical that the rationale behind the use of exposure therapy be explained carefully because without a clear understanding of and faith in the rationale, participants might not be able to tolerate the intense and often emotionally upsetting side effects. Furthermore, if the increase in symptoms that often accompanies the initial phase of treatment is not normalized, participants may be more likely to interpret their distress as an indication that the treatment is failing and may terminate treatment before the disturbing material is successfully processed. For these reasons, the rationale was reinforced throughout the treatment. In addition to providing participants with the treatment rationale, it was deemed important to educate others who were significant in the participants' lives as well, especially regarding the expected temporary worsening of symptoms.

During the first session, a neutral VR environment that does not contain threat cues was demonstrated to familiarize participants with the VR technology and to teach them how to navigate within it. In the final part of the first session, the veteran was taught a breathing exercise for stress management and was asked to practice this exercise daily. During the second and third sessions, the participant was exposed to one of the Virtual Vietnam environments. During these initial exposure sessions, the veteran was encouraged to acclimate to the environment and only describe the memories that were triggered by being there.

After the participant was somewhat familiar with the Vietnam environment, he was asked to focus on the specific traumatic memory that he wanted to address in therapy. The participant was asked to describe this incident as if it were occurring in the present (e.g., " I see the enemy coming"). As the participant described the traumatic event, the therapist tracked what was being said and provided associated visual and auditory stimuli. This added a level of reality to the participant's recounting, which aided their ability to connect to and stay with the traumatic memories being described. Whenever possible, the therapist encouraged participants to remain with the traumatic memory until their resulting anxiety was substantially reduced. The therapist's goal was to provide the optimum level of stimulation without overwhelming the participant.

Following the completion of VRE, participants were given a post-treatment assessment. PTSD symptoms were again measured with the test battery, so that the post-treatment scores could be easily compared with the participants' pre-treatment scores on this measure. In addition, follow-up assessments were performed at three and six months. A comparison of the scores obtained at these follow-up times and the patients' pre-and post-treatment scores allowed the authors to determine whether any therapeutic gains made during or immediately following VRE were maintained over time.

Description of a Typical VRE Session

A typical VRE session started with an assessment of the participants' current mental state and their response to treatment up to that point. This was done to monitor participants' progress in therapy, to assess for any adverse treatment effects, and to determine if the participant could tolerate a more intense exposure at that point in time. If the therapist determined that it was not in the participant's best interest to participate in VRE during that session, then the remainder of the session was spent addressing whatever concern(s) had been raised. If, on the other hand, the therapist determined that the participant would benefit from continued exposure experiences, then a discussion ensued concerning what would occur during the exposure part of that session. The therapist determined whether to continue exposing the participant to the level of stimulation that was used during the previous session, to increase the exposure's intensity, or to decrease it depending on the input provided during the course of this discussion. This process generally took 15 to 20 minutes to complete. Once the therapist and the participant agreed on what would happen, the participant put on the Head Mounted Display and the exposure phase began. This phase typically lasted for between 30 and 45 minutes.

As stated previously, the goal of a VR exposure is to provide enough stimuli to keep the participant engaged in the traumatic memory without overwhelming him. This goal was accomplished by carefully monitoring participants' behavior during the exposure experience. Therefore, while in a VR environment, participants remained in constant contact with the therapist. The therapist was able to see and hear everything that the participant did, using a separate computer monitor and speakers. The therapist communicated with the patient through a microphone that is patched into the HMD. As part of the monitoring process, participants are asked to provide a SUDS rating at five-minute intervals during the exposure phase of a session. This rating was used in conjunction with the therapist's clinical judgment to ensure that participants received an optimal level of VR stimulation. Since some patients tended to underreport SUDS scores, clinical judgement was needed to interpret how each patient was utilizing the SUDS. In addition to the SUDS rating, the therapist watched for changes in the participant's body language (e.g., cringing) and voice (e.g., halting or stammering) that may be indicative of how the participant was responding to the treatment. Furthermore, the content of the participant's comments was also considered in determining whether an appropriate level of stimulation was being used. For example, a comment suggesting that the environment did not seem real enough would indicate an insufficient level of external stimulation, while a comment suggesting that the participant was feeling overwhelmed by the experience would indicate a need to decrease the intensity of the external stimuli being presented.

After the VR exposure phase had concluded, participants were asked to describe their exposure experience and provide feedback to the therapist. Often individuals became physically and emotionally aroused while in the VR environment. These debriefings provided participants with an opportunity to calm down and to discuss their experience of the exposure phase. This process took approximately 15 minutes to complete. Provisions were made for additional time to be available if necessary, although this was rarely needed. An audio-cassette recording was made of the exposure portion of each VRE session. Participants were instructed to take the cassette home and use it to practice imaginal exposure daily between sessions. Providing participants with the means to engage in repeated exposures to the traumatic material between sessions was found to benefit recovery, as patients often felt encouraged to continue treatment by the decrease in emotional responses that occurred with repeated exposures to the same tape recording.

Termination of treatment. VRE concluded when the participant was able to describe the traumatic event in great detail, while being exposed to intense external stimuli, without significant emotional discomfort. Participants should be able to recognize a memory as being "sad" or "horrible" without feeling as if they are reliving the experience every time they recall the associated event. We have found that this objective was typically reached in 10 sessions. It also seemed that patients who had never discussed their Vietnam experiences before and/or who had a high degree of combat exposure required additional sessions to reach this point.

RESULTS

Table 1 contains the mean ± SD values for outcome measures at pretreatment, post-treatment, and the 3- and 6-month follow-up. There were statistically significant reductions in clinician rated symptoms as measured by the total CAPS score, the primary outcome measure, on all three post-treatment assessments (see Table 1). Two patients had CAPS scores on their immediate post-treatment assessments that were higher than their pretreatment scores (+41% and +13%, respectively). All patients' scores on the 3- and 6-month follow-up assessments were below their pretreatment scores (range −15 to −67%). There were significant reductions in the avoidance and arousal subscales of the CAPS on all post-treatment assessments and in the intrusion subscale on 3- and 6-month assessments. In sharp contrast to the rebound effect found in many studies of Vietnam veterans, the continued decrease in total average CAPS scores over the three post treatment assessments indicates that patients continued to improve for months after treatment was terminated.

Patient's self-reported intrusion symptoms as measured by the IES were significantly lower on all post-treatment assessments. The total IES scores and the avoidance subscale scores were significantly lower on the 3- and 6-month assessments (see Table 1). One explanation for the contrast between the insignificant change in the intrusion score on the CAPS and the significant reduction in the intrusion score on the IES

TABLE 1. Summary of Outcome Measures at Baseline (Pretreatment, and 3- and 6-Months Follow-Up)

	Baseline[b] (N = 14*)	Post-Treatment (N = 14)		3 Month Follow-Up (N = 8)		6 Month Follow-Up (N = 11)	
		Value[b]	p[c]	Value[b]	p[c]	Value[b]	p[c]
CAPS[a]							
Total	72.57 ± 16.18	59.64 ± 17.77	.0140	55.13 ± 14.38	.0027	50.91 ± 17.24	.0001
% Change from baseline, mean (Range)	...	−17 (+41 to −51)	...	−30 (−13 to −52)	...	−32 (−15 to −67)	...
Intrusion	18.43 ± 6.66	16.36 ± 7.07	.3852	11.50 ± 6.89	.0412	12.00 ± 4.15	.0056
Avoidance	29.36 ± 8.65	20.71 ± 7.49	.0158	21.00 ± 7.50	.0023	18.73 ± 8.63	.0008
Arousal	24.79 ± 4.90	22.57 ± 9.80	.0287	22.63 ± 4.00	.0245	20.18 ± 6.35	.0011
Impact of Event Scale							
Total	45.29 ± 10.43	34.50 ± 20.80	.1033	19.88 ± 11.32	.0020	30.82 ± 16.61	.0172
Intrusion	22.50 ± 6.05	16.43 ± 8.22	.0323	8.88 ± 7.22	.0004	13.73 ± 9.64	.0238
Avoidance	22.79 ± 8.14	18.07 ± 14.51	.2642	11.00 ± 4.90	.0170	16.18 ± 9.12	.0303
BDI	24.86 ± 9.70	21.14 ± 8.18	.0454	24.25 ± 9.53	.2631	18.45 ± 9.49	.0043

[a] Abbreviation....
[b] Values shown as mean ± SD unless noted otherwise
[c] p Values vs. baseline
* 9 of these subjects already reported on in Rothbaum et al. (2001)

is that the CAPS intrusion subscale is an overall measure of re-experiencing symptoms whereas the IES intrusion subscale is a measure of re-experiencing symptoms related to the specific event that was the focus of the VRE treatment. It is not uncommon for a veteran to report that talking about the details of a specific event in Vietnam led to a temporary increase in intrusive memories about other war experiences. It may be true that VRE produced an immediate and sustained decrease in the re-experiencing symptoms related to the events that were the specific focus of treatment while a change in the overall degree of war-related re-experiencing symptoms took more time to develop.

Symptoms of depression, as measured by the BDI, may have also been affected by VRE. There was a statistically significant reduction in the BDI scores from pretreatment to immediate post-treatment assessment that was not maintained on the 3-month follow-up evaluation. However, the reduction found on the 6-month follow-up assessment is both statistically and clinically significant (see Table 1).

It seems clear that VRE produced statistically significant reductions in the PTSD symptoms that were both clinically significant and lasting in the combined sample of 14 patients who completed at least one post-treatment assessment in the Atlanta open trials. Consistent with many other exposure-based studies, patients continued to improve even after the treatment was completed; thus, the full effects of the treatment are not apparent without follow-up assessments (Foa, Rothbaum, Riggs, & Murdock, 1991).

Overall, the results of VRE have been encouraging. Of the 14 participants who completed VRE treatment and attended at least one post-treatment assessment, only two reported significant increases in PTSD symptoms during the course of treatment while the rest reported only mild increases in symptoms. All responses to VRE treatment were easily handled on an outpatient basis. All 14 patients showed reductions in PTSD symptoms compared to baseline by the 3-month follow-up assessment. These gains were maintained in 10 of the 11 patients who completed the 6-month follow-up assessment. In six of these patients, the CAPS scores continued to decline between the immediate post-treatment assessment and the 6-month assessment.

CASE STUDIES

Two case studies were selected to illustrate the benefits of VRE therapy in the treatment of veterans with war-related PTSD. The first is a typical case and the second one is a veteran who experienced significant increases in symptoms during VRE yet obviously benefited substantially from this treatment.

Case 1: Caught in the Middle

Mr. D is a 56-year-old Caucasian Army veteran who served three weeks in Vietnam before being wounded in combat and medically evacuated. He has a 100% service-connected disability for PTSD. VRE treatment focused on his traumatic memories of being wounded while driving a fuel truck in 1967. The traumatic events occurred 34 years prior to treatment. The trauma began when a bullet pierced his windshield and knocked the helmet off his head. Seconds later, an explosion knocked his truck on its side, driving the back of the engine into the cab compartment. Mr. D was wounded by gunshots in both feet, suffered a head laceration, and received numerous other injuries. Despite limited mobility, he managed to climb out of the cab, only to find that he was caught in the crossfire between American and enemy forces. Mr. D had no means of defending himself and was forced to play dead when a group of enemy soldiers came within ten feet of him. Several hours later, he was rescued and flown to a field hospital where he witnessed a friend bleed to death on the stretcher next to him.

Prior to VRE treatment, Mr. D told the therapist his "story" of being wounded. The therapist commented to Mr. D that he had told his story with no real emotion. Mr. D reported that he had told the story many times over the years, but indicated that he felt very little emotional connection to the event. Mr. D received a total of twelve VRE sessions. As Mr. D repeated his story in VRE, he became much more emotional. He recalled many details he had forgotten, and experienced numerous body memories (physical sensations that occur while recounting traumatic memories that are similar to the actual physical sensations that occurred during the event), such as his legs hurting where he was wounded. These body memories and the degree of emotionality dissipated as therapy progressed and Mr. D processed this traumatic event.

During VRE, the landing zone environment was used. Although this environment lacks trucks or images of a convoy, the audio input was similar enough to Mr. D's experience to assist him in partially reliving these events. For example, as he described suddenly having his helmet shot off his head, the therapist turned on the enemy machine-gun fire. Similarly, when he mentioned the explosion that turned his truck on its side, the land mine sound was triggered and a bright flash was activated.

While Mr. D described being on the ground caught in the crossfire, the enemy machine-gun fire, mortar explosions, rocket explosions, screaming, and battle ambience (a firefight in the distance) were turned on. As he described the enemy withdrawing these sounds faded away as the therapist lowered the volume and after a while turned off the combat stimuli. Furthermore, the sounds of a helicopter taking off and landing were used to simulate Mr. D's flight to a field hospital. Finally, when he told about witnessing his friend bleeding to death, the sounds of helicopters coming, landing, powering down their engines, and the sounds of helicopters taking off were used due to their similarity to sounds in a field hospital.

On his immediate post-treatment assessment, Mr. D's CAPS score was 51% lower than on his pre-treatment (93 at pre-treatment versus 46 at post-treatment). There were reductions in all three-symptom clusters of PTSD: re-experiencing (32 pre-treatment versus 14 post-treatment], arousal (31 pre-treatment versus 22 post-treatment) and avoidance/numbing (30 pre-treatment versus 10 post-treatment). These reductions were maintained at the 3-month follow-up assessment (CAPS score at 3-month follow-up = 45). At the 6-month follow-up, Mr. D reported an increase in the avoidance/numbing symptoms (25). However, his overall CAPS score (63) was still 32% lower than at his pre-treatment assessment. It is possible that the increase in avoidance/numbing symptoms reported by Mr. D was due, in part, to his relocating across the country shortly after finishing treatment, since his relocation increased his isolation and disrupted his continued PTSD treatment. When questioned about whether or not he would recommend this treatment to other veterans, Mr. D stated, "While it is not for everyone, I would swear by this treatment."

Case 2: Rip Van Winkle

Mr. J is a 53-year-old African American Marine veteran who experienced heavy combat exposure in Vietnam and was wounded in action. VRE treatment focused on memories of the night his base camp was overrun and temporarily taken over by enemy troops. During this night in 1968, many Marines lost their lives. Mr. J barely escaped being killed several times, was wounded, and witnessed other Marines being executed as they tried to surrender to the enemy. This event occurred 33 years prior to VRE treatment.

Mr. J had 20 VRE sessions using the landing zone environment. During exposure, Mr. J reported many body memories, particularly in the leg where he had been wounded. These body memories dissipated as therapy progressed. VRE started in daylight as his squad prepared for the night. Next, the darkness mode was turned on. Mr. J then described how the night was quiet until his friend threw out a flare. Suddenly, they discovered that a massive number of the enemy were just a few feet away. At that point in his narrative, a soundless white flash was used to emulate the flare. As Mr. J described the attack, the therapist initiated the sights and sounds of enemy machine-gun fire, mortar explosions, screaming, land mine explosions, and battle ambience in accordance with his description. Frequent white flashes without explosions were used to simulate flares being launched. Towards the end of the exposure, the sounds of helicopters were used to simulate the gun ships that flew overhead at the end of the attack. Daylight with heavy fog was restored near the end of the exposure. During the last few minutes of the exposure, the sounds of helicopters taking off and landing were used to simulate the flight of Mr. J as he was flown from the base camp to a field hospital.

The empirical results of Mr. J's VRE treatment were mixed. His post-treatment CAPS score was 13% higher than his pre-treatment total CAPS score (68 pre-treatment versus 77 post-treatment). This overall elevation was primarily due to a reported increase in re-experiencing symptoms (14 pre-treatment versus 31 post-treatment). With time, however, Mr. J's PTSD symptoms began to decrease. His 3-month follow-up total CAPS score of 57 was 16% lower than his pretreatment score and his 6-month post treatment CAPS score of 44 was 35% lower. At the 6 months follow-up assessment, Mr. J reported a level of re-experiencing symptoms that was just slightly below his pre-treatment level (13). Therefore, VRE did not produce significant reductions in Mr. J's re-experiencing PTSD symptoms, but it did foster remarkable reductions in the avoidance/numbing and arousal symptom clusters, as well as in his overall level of symptomology

Mr. J also reported making dramatic lifestyle changes following the completion of his VRE treatment. Prior to VRE, Mr. J reported having been unable to discuss anything related to Vietnam for over thirty years. He became angry and withdrew from others if they asked him about the war. According to Mr. J, as he progressed in VRE therapy he was better able to tolerate thinking and talking about Vietnam. In addition, he reported being better able to deal with memories of Vietnam when they were triggered. He indicated that others recognized this change as well. For example, Mr. J's mother showed him a box she had kept hidden from him for over three decades. The box contained letters he had written from Vietnam, photos of him in the service, and an article from the local newspaper about the time he was wounded. She told him that she had never shown the box to him before because he became so angry whenever the topic of Vietnam arose. Mr. J was able to calmly go through the box and view each item without becoming emotionally overwhelmed; he was even able to share the content of this box with his adult daughter. In addition, he started participating in weekly group therapy sessions, which he said were very rewarding.

Mr. J was also able to attend his son's wedding. This was significant because Mr. J had generally avoided crowds and had never attended a church wedding and reception. He did not attend his daughter's wedding or the weddings of his siblings. Mr. J reported that his son was so pleased that he asked him to serve as best man. Other changes reported by Mr. J included feeling more comfortable going out at night, developing a close friendship with another male for the first time since the war, attending his daughter's basketball game, and a decrease in his re-experiencing of the specific traumatic events that were the focus of VRE. Prior to VRE, Mr. J's main defense was to consume himself with work. Following treatment, however, he regretted all the years he had lost with his family by working 16-hour days and felt no desire to continue working such long hours. Overall, then, Mr. J reported experiencing a better quality of life since the completion of his VRE therapy. In a way, it is as if Mr. J had awakened from a prolonged nightmare, and became able to participate much more in the positive aspects of life from which he had withdrawn for over thirty years.

DISCUSSION

VR is a revolutionary technology that gives patients a strong sense of being present in a computer-generated environment. In VR, the therapist can control every sight and sound in a virtual environment on a moment-to-moment basis. VR opens up a new means of providing exposure therapy that has many advantages over traditional methods. With VR, patients can be exposed to feared stimuli, in order to become desensitized to these stimuli, with the therapist having complete control over the intensity and duration of this exposure. VR exposure therapy can be safer, more convenient, and more practical than in vivo exposure and may be more effective than imaginal exposure with some patient populations. Due to these advantages, VR has been used to successfully treat phobias (Anderson et al., 2000). Based on the effectiveness of VR with phobias, it has also been hypothesized that VR may be used to treat PTSD (Rothbaum et al., 1999). An analysis that combined the data from two open trials with Vietnam veterans at the Atlanta VA Medical Center indicates that VRE can produce clinically significant and lasting reductions in PTSD symptoms with some Vietnam veterans. This is particularly noteworthy because Vietnam veterans have been found to be one of the most treatment resistant PTSD patient populations (Foa et al., 2000).

Additional support for the utility of VRE can be found in two recently published case reports. One was of a veteran at the Boston VA Medical Center (Rothbaum, Ruef, Litz, Han, & Hodges, 2003) who showed significant reductions in PTSD symptoms at the 6-month follow-up assessment. The other is of a successfully treated civilian survivor of the September 11 terrorist attack in New York. In this study, a 26-year-old female survivor who had not benefited from imaginal exposure had a dramatic (90%) reduction in PTSD symptoms after six one-hour VRE sessions using an environment specifically designed to simulate elements of the attack on the World Trade Center (Difede & Hoffman, 2002).

Although caution is needed when interpreting the significance of uncontrolled case studies, we believe that it is reasonable to suggest that VRE may be an important new tool in the treatment of PTSD. For example, the US military already uses VR to prepare troops for combat. There may come a time when this same equipment will be used to routinely treat soldiers who are suffering from PTSD symptoms while they are still in the service. Clearly, VRE is likely to be a fruitful area for further research, and controlled studies are urgently needed to investigate this new treatment modality. In the absence of controlled studies, it is premature to draw any conclusions about the utility of VRE for PTSD. We believe that the positive findings so far suggest that VRE could become a cost efficient and effective means of providing treatment to a variety of PTSD patient populations in the future.

REFERENCES

American Psychiatric Association. (1994). *Diagnostic and statistical manual of mental disorders* (4th Ed.). Washington, DC: Author.

Anderson, P. L., Rothbaum, B. O., & Hodges, L. (2001). Virtual reality: Using the virtual world to improve quality of life in the real world. *Bulletin of the Menninger Clinic, 65,* 78-91.

Beck, A. T., Ward, C. H., Mendelsohn, M., Mock, J., & Erbaugh, J. (1961). An inventory for measuring depression. *Archives of General Psychiatry, 4*, 561-571.

Blake, D. D., Weathers, F., Nagy, L. M., Kaloupek, D. G., Klauminzer, G., Charney, D. S. et al. (1990). A clinician rating scale for assessing current and lifetime PTSD: The CAPS-1. *The Behavior Therapist, 13*, 187-188.

Boudewyns, P. A. (1994). Direct therapeutic exposure: A learning theory-based approach to the treatment of PTSD. In L. Hyer (Ed.), *Trauma victim: Theoretical issues and practical suggestions* (pp. 523-568). Muncie, IN: Accelerated Development Inc.

Boudewyns, P. A., Hyer, L., Woods, M. G., Harrison, W. R., & McCrame, E. (1990). PTSD among Vietnam Veterans: An early look at treatment outcome using direct therapeutic exposure. *Journal of Traumatic Stress, 3*, 359-398.

Cooper, N. A., & Clum, G. A. (1989). Imaginal flooding as a supplementary treatment for PTSD in combat veterans: A controlled study. *Behavior Therapy, 20*, 381-391.

Devilly, G. J., Spence, S. H., & Rapee, R. M. (1998). Statistical and reliable change with eye movement desensitization and reprocessing: Treating trauma within a veteran population. *Behavior Therapy, 29*(3), 435-455.

Difede, J., & Hoffman, H. G. (2002). Virtual reality exposure therapy for World Trade Center post-traumatic stress disorder: A case report. *Cyberpsychology & Behavior, 5*, 529-535.

Fairbank, J. A., Gross, R. T., & Keane, T. M. (1983). Treatment of posttraumatic stress disorder: Evaluation of outcome with a behavioral code. *Behavior Modification, 7*, 557-568.

Foa, E. B., Keane, T. M., & Friedman, M. J. (Eds.) (2000). *Effective treatment for PTSD: Practice guidelines from the International Society of Traumatic Stress Studies.* New York: Guilford Press.

Foa, E. B., & Kozak, M. J. (1986). Emotional processing of fear: Exposure to corrective information. *Psychological Bulletin, 99*, 20-35.

Foa, E. B., & Rothbaum, B. O. (1998). *Treating the trauma of rape: Cognitive-behavioral therapy for PTSD.* New York: Guilford Press.

Foa, E. B., Rothbaum, B. O., Riggs, D., & Murdock, T. (1991). Treatment of posttraumatic stress disorder in rape victims: A comparison between cognitive-behavioral procedures and counseling. *Journal of Consulting and Clinical Psychology, 59*, 715-723.

Foa, E. B., Steketee, G., & Rothbaum, B. (1989). Behavioral/cognitive conceptualizations of post-traumatic stress disorder. *Behavior Therapy, 20*, 155-176.

Fontana, A., Rosenheck, R., & Spencer, H. (1993). *The long journey home III: The third progress report on the Department of Veterans Affairs Specialized PTSD programs.* West Haven, CT: Northeast Program Evaluation Center, Evaluation Division of the National Center for PTSD, Department of Veterans Affairs Medical Center.

Frueh, B. C., Turner, S. M., Beidel, D. C., Mirabella, R. F., & Jones, W. J. (1996). Trauma management therapy: A preliminary evaluation of a multicomponent behavioral treatment for chronic combat-related PTSD. *Behaviour Research & Therapy, 34*, 533-543

Glynn, S. M., Eth, S., Eugenia, R. T., Foy, D. W., Urbaitis, M., Boxer, L. et al. (1999). A test of behavioral family therapy to augment exposure for combat-related posttraumatic stress disorder. *Journal of Consulting and Clinical Psychology, 67,* 243-251.

Hammarberg, M., & Silver, S. M. (1994). Outcome of treatment for post-traumatic stress disorder in a primary care unit serving Vietnam veterans. *Journal of Traumatic Stress, 7*(2), 195-216.

Horowitz, M. J., Wilner, N., & Alvarez, W. (1979). Impact of event scale: A measure of subjective distress. *Psychosomatic Medicine, 41,* 207-218.

Johnson, C. H., Gilmore, J. D., & Shenoy, R. Z. (1982). Use of a flooding procedure in the treatment of a stress-related anxiety disorder. *Journal of Behavior Therapy and Experimental Psychiatry, 13,* 235-237.

Johnson, D. R., Rosenheck, R., Fontana, A., Lubin, H., Charney, M. D., & Southwick, M. D. (1996). Outcome of intensive inpatient treatment for combat-related posttraumatic stress disorder. *American Journal of Psychiatry, 153,* 771-777.

Kaplan, D. M., Smith, T., & Coons, J. (1995). A validity study of the subjective unit of discomfort (SUD) score. *Measurement & Evaluation in Counseling & Development, 27,* 195-199.

Keane, T. M., Caddell, J. M., & Taylor, K. L. (1988). The Mississippi scale for combat-related PTSD: Three studies in reliability and validity. *Journal of Consulting and Clinical Psychology, 56,* 85-90.

Keane, T. M., Fairbank, J. A., Caddell, J. M., & Zimmering, R. T. (1989). Implosive (flooding) therapy reduces symptoms for PTSD in Vietnam combat veterans. *Behavior Therapy, 20,* 245-260.

Keane, T. M., & Kaloupek, D. G. (1982). Imaginal flooding in the treatment of post-traumatic stress disorder. *Journal of Consulting and Clinical Psychology, 50,* 138-140.

Lipke, H. J., & Botkin, A. L. (1992). Case studies of eye movement desensitization and reprocessing (EMDR) with chronic post-traumatic stress disorder. *Psychotherapy, Theory, Research, Practice, Training, 29*(4), 591-595.

Macklin, M., Metzger, L. J., Lasko, N. B., Berry, N. J., Orr, S. P., & Pittman, R. K. (2000). Five-year follow-up study of eye movement desensitization and reprocessing therapy for combat-related posttraumatic stress disorder. *Comprehensive Psychiatry, 41*(1), 24-27.

Rosenheck, F. A., Spencer, H., & Gray, S. (2002). *The long journey home X: Treatment of posttraumatic stress disorder in the Department of Veterans Affairs: Fiscal Year 2001 service delivery and performance.* West Haven, CT: Northeast Program Evaluation Center.

Rothbaum, B. O., Hodges, L., Alarcon, R., Ready, D., Sharhar, F., Pair, J. et al. (1999). Virtual reality exposure therapy for PTSD Vietnam veterans: A case study. *Journal of Traumatic Stress, 12,* 263-271.

Rothbaum, B. O., Hodges, L. F., Ready, D., Graap, K., & Alarcon, M. D. (2001). Virtual reality exposure therapy for Vietnam veterans with posttraumatic stress disorder. *Journal of Clinical Psychiatry, 62,* 617-622.

Rothbaum, B. O., Meadows, E. A., Resick, P, & Foy, D. W. (2000). Cognitive-behavioral therapy. In E. B. Foa, T. M. Keane, & M. J. Friedman (Eds.), *Effective treatment for PTSD: Practice guidelines from the International Society of Traumatic Stress Studies* (pp. 60-83). New York: Guilford Press.

Rothbaum, B. O., Ruef, A. M., Litz, B. T., Han, H., & Hodges, L. (2003). Virtual reality Exposure therapy of combat-related PTSD: A case study using psychophysiological indicators of outcome. *Journal of Cognitive Psychotherapy, 17*, 163-177.

Schnurr, P. P, Friedman, M. J., Foy, D. W., Shea, M. T., Hsieh, F. Y., Lavori, P. W. et al. (2003). Randomized trial of trauma-focused group therapy for posttraumatic stress disorder: Results from a Department of Veterans Affairs cooperative study. *Archives of General Psychiatry, 60*, 481-489.

Shapiro, F. (1999). Eye movement desensitization and reprocessing (EMDR) and anxiety disorders: Clinical and research implications of an integrated psychotherapy treatment. *Journal of Anxiety Disorders, 13*, 35-67.

van der Kolk, B.A., Dreyfuss, D., Michaels, M., Shera, D., Berkowitz, R., Fisher, R. et al. (1994). Fluoxetine in posttraumatic stress disorder. *Journal of Clinical Psychiatry, 146*, 517-222.

Weathers, F. W., & Litz, B. T. (1994). Psychometric properties of the Clinician Administered PTSD scale. *PTSD Research Quarterly, 5*, 2-6.

Weiss, D. S., Marmar, C. R., Schlenger, W. E., Fairbank, J. A., Jordan, B. K., Hough, R. L. et al. (1992). The prevalence of lifetime and partial post-traumatic stress disorder in Vietnam theater veterans. *Journal of Traumatic Stress, 5*, 365-376.

Zadecki, J. (1999). PTSD treatment outcome: A conference report. *Veterans Health System Journal, 7*, 15-22.

Technologies to Lessen the Distress of Autism

Ron Oberleitner
James Ball
Dan Gillette
Robert Naseef
B. Hudnall Stamm

SUMMARY. This article explores aspects of autism that make it a potential traumatic stressor for family members, and may put them at risk for Posttraumatic Stress Disorder (PTSD) and/or its sub-syndromal variants. It also surveys current trends in autism, including the growing number of families affected by autism. Because PTSD and its sub-syndromes can benefit from prevention or at least bolstering the resources of the person and their social support system, this article will then focus on relevant technology trends being used to mediate or ameliorate aspects of living with autism. This technology includes telehealth, distance education, information technology, video-conferencing, and computer software. *[Article copies available for a fee from The Haworth Document Delivery Service: 1-800-HAWORTH. E-mail address: <docdelivery@haworthpress.com> Website: <http://www.HaworthPress.com> © 2006 by The Haworth Press, Inc. All rights reserved.]*

Address correspondence to Ron Oberleitner, P.O. Box 1348, Princeton, NJ 08540.
The opinions or assertions contained herein are the private ones of the authors, and are not to be considered as official or reflecting the views of the authors' institutions.

[Haworth co-indexing entry note]: "Technologies to Lessen the Distress of Autism." Oberleitner, Ron et al. Co-published simultaneously in *Journal of Aggression, Maltreatment & Trauma* (The Haworth Maltreatment & Trauma Press, an imprint of The Haworth Press, Inc.) Vol. 12, No. 1/2, 2006, pp. 221-242; and: *Trauma Treatment Techniques: Innovative Trends* (ed: Jacqueline Garrick, and Mary Beth Williams) The Haworth Maltreatment & Trauma Press, an imprint of The Haworth Press, Inc., 2006, pp. 221-242. Single or multiple copies of this article are available for a fee from The Haworth Document Delivery Service [1-800-HAWORTH, 9:00 a.m. - 5:00 p.m. (EST). E-mail address: docdelivery@haworthpress.com].

Available online at http://www.haworthpress.com/web/JAMT
© 2006 by The Haworth Press, Inc. All rights reserved.
doi:10.1300/J146v12n01_12

KEYWORDS. Autism, telehealth, telemedicine, traumatic stress, PTSD

Families dealing with special needs children face amazing challenges. Giving birth to a severely developmentally delayed or handicapped baby has been referred to as a trauma (Stern & Bruschweiler-Stern, 1998). It is a crisis that is emotionally staggering, and it obliterates the hopes and fantasies of the pregnancy. For families who have children diagnosed with autism, one of the most devastating and misunderstood of childhood development disorders, they frequently experience additional layers of distress because of the unique nature of the syndrome. For example, one parent of a child with autism stated,

> Just hearing the Autism word was a trauma to me at first. It took me a long time before I could use my son's name and the "A" word in the same sentence. Now, finally, I feel that using it empowers me. It takes the stigma away from my son personally and puts it where it belongs, on a neurological condition.

Historically, autism has been relatively unknown by the mainstream medical community, yet recent estimates show between 0.5 and 1.5 million Americans suffer from an autism spectrum disorder (Autism Society of America, 2002). Typically, autism causes irreparable neurological damage affecting the child's ability to communicate and socialize adequately, and triggering behaviors that range from compulsions to painful responses to normal stimuli, along with self-harming or violent behavior towards others. Autism is a lifelong disability with no known cure and no standard medical treatments. Many proposed treatments are poorly substantiated in terms of effectiveness and are difficult to document, except anecdotally.

While most families adapt to the unique challenges of having a member with autism, they generally experience loss and face ongoing autism-related stress. In some cases, living with autism itself produces situations in which there is danger to the person with autism or his or her family members. In these cases, Posttraumatic Stress Disorder (PTSD) may emerge. Whether or not the person with autism will, or even can, develop PTSD is poorly documented and poorly understood (Newman, Christopher, & Berry, 2000) and deserves additional study. The risk to parents and family members has not been discussed in the literature and is a focus of this paper. This risk can come either by being inadvertently hurt by the person with autism as a result of an aspect of their disease, or witnessing the person with autism in danger as a result of the person not understanding the danger of a situation. Another parent stated:

> Just the other day, Jimmy stepped out of the street-side door of the car and began to run directly into the street without looking. I grabbed him just as a minivan put on the brakes. The brakes didn't screech, but the driver looked badly shaken. I held Jimmy to me with all my force. If only my mother love could protect him! My friend who was picking up her child at my house held my hand–hers was shaking. Jimmy seemed completely unfazed by any of this.

This article explores aspects of autism that make it a potential traumatic stressor for family members,[1] and may put them at risk for Posttraumatic Stress Disorder (PTSD) and/or its sub-syndromal variants. It also surveys current trends in autism, including the growing number of families affected by autism. Because PTSD and its sub-syndromes can benefit from prevention or at least bolstering the resources of the person and their social support system, this article will then focus on relevant technology trends being used to mediate or ameliorate aspects of living with autism. This technology includes telehealth, distance education, information technology, video-conferencing, and computer software.

AUTISM DEFINED

Autism is a devastating, pervasive developmental disability that usually appears between 15 and 20 months of age (Akshoomoff, 2000). Although all people with autism do not present exactly the same symptoms and deficits, the disease is characterized by social, communication, motor, and sensory problems that frequently create distressing behaviors. The diagnostic criteria address impairment in three areas: (a) social interaction, (b) impaired communication, and (c) stereotypic and repetitive behaviors (American Psychiatric Association [APA], 2000). Impaired social interaction includes reduced eye contact; failure to develop peer relationships; absence of spontaneous joy or interest; and lack of social or emotional reciprocity. The second diagnostic criterion, impaired communication, involves delay in or failure to develop spoken language; impaired ability to have a conversation; stereotyped, repetitive, idiosyncratic language; and lack of symbolic play. The final criterion is stereotypic and repetitive behavior, which includes preoccupation, inflexibility and rigidity, motor mannerisms such as hand flapping and spinning, and preoccupations with parts of objects.

There is a broad spectrum of behavioral manifestations upon which the diagnosis of autism is made. Also, there are related and heterogeneous abnormalities responsible for the complexity in the way this disorder presents itself. Understanding the individual profile of the child is crucial to developing the most efficacious treatment plan (Greenspan & Weider, 1999).

While some children with autism will never speak, most will progress through many familiar developmental milestones. Some have the beginnings of speech in early development and then lose it. These children may regain speech, or they will likely be able to develop some form of communication through gestures, signs, or picture exchange. Because autism remains throughout one's life, they may not be able to marry or live independently, resulting in long-term demands on caretakers. People with autism may have symptoms that include sleeplessness, obsessions, hyperactivity, and even self-injuring behavior. These behaviors put the person with autism at risk and pose severe challenges, including isolation, for their caretakers. Further, how the condition of each individual progresses is largely dependent on the interaction between his or her innate factors and the individual's caregivers and treatment modalities.

HOW AUTISM PUTS THE FAMILY AT RISK

Parents report feeling more relaxed when they have enough resources to help their child (Seligman & Darling, 1997). The constant and evolving struggles of the family who must cope with chronic depletion of resources make family members vulnerable to a variety of problems. These problems may require intervention, and may diminish when the family is successful in finding concrete help for the child.

Preexisting vulnerabilities may rekindle with the stress of caring for a child with autism, precipitating new clinical episodes. One of the most draining problems families deal with is hyperactivity and the lack of sleep a child with autism may experience. Sleep can be a major issue for people with autism; for example, after only two hours' sleep, a child affected by autism may be up and on the move for the next day (Durand, 1998). For weary parents, this lack of sleep can challenge the family's coping and exacerbate physical and mental risk factors.

In addition to the feelings of loss a family may feel learning that their child has autism, the child's various behaviors and their unpredictability cause considerable stress for families (Bristol, 1984). Many children with autism cry and tantrum incessantly, break things, injure themselves, and shriek at high pitches. These behaviors may arise because the child cannot communicate or experiences pain caused by his or her environment. In some cases, the child's behavior may incorporate a very clear life threat such as running out of the house into traffic, into pools or lakes, or even up high-tension towers. They may break windows or dart into a neighbor's house to search for items they are obsessed with, such as video players, remote controls, and televisions. Just to ensure that the autistic child will not escape, families may essentially barricade themselves into their home, putting the whole family at risk should they need to evacuate the home, such as in the case of a fire. This environment of captivity, designed to gain at least a modicum of safety and control for the family, has been identified by Herman (1992) as a major contributor to long-term, complex traumatic stress. In addition, these highly-charged environments present multiple risk factors for family violence, a commonly recognized precipitant of traumatic stress.

The general understanding of trauma assigns a variety of meanings to the word, but according to the *Diagnostic and Statistical Manual* (APA, 2000) definition there must be a personal experience of an event that involves actual or threatened death to self or another or threat to one's physical integrity (PTSD Criterion A1) accompanied by a response of intense fear, helplessness, or horror (Criterion A2). A person may be the direct target of the event, or they may experience the event by witnessing or by learning about such an event that has happened to a family member or close associate (APA, 2000). The symptom clusters that make up the diagnosis of PTSD include intrusion, avoidance, and hyperarousal.

A hallmark of traumatic stress is that it is an overwhelming experience that affects mind and body and impacts people's ability to think and make sense out of current experiences (van der Kolk, McFarlane, & Weisaeth, 1996). Stress and extreme stress threaten one's sense of coherence (SOC) (Antonovsky, 1979, 1987). SOC includes comprehensibility of how ordered and consistent one's world is. It also includes manageability (e.g., one's ability to mobilize resources to cope) and meaningfulness of one's experiences. Extremely stressful events not only challenge SOC, they may color one's interpretation of new experiences such that the stressor is the pervasive organizing schema of one's life (Jannoff-Bulman, 1992; Stamm, 1999a, 1999b).

It can be difficult *not* to react to autism-related experiences with fear, helplessness, or horror because of the dramatic characteristics of the disorder and its chronic nature. Just as the family overcomes one crisis, another crisis takes its place, intensifying as the child grows older, larger, and stronger. For example, one parent of a child with autism stated:

> And there are other traumas like Jimmy hitting me, especially as he gets bigger. It physically hurts more, but I'm also not able to restrain him effectively. Now when he yells he's gotten a lot louder. It brings up all of the years of being hit and yelled at by him. When Jimmy obstructs a turnstile, or lays down on the floor of a bookstore, the trauma there is more looking into the future. I fear he'll have a run-in with the police, or even be shot for resisting arrest.

When the chronic challenges of autism include dangerousness, people in the family may meet Criterion A1 and A2 of PTSD. There is no research available of how common this may be, but certainly in some extreme cases, people may experience the characteristic symptoms of PTSD that include three symptom clusters: (Criterion B) intrusion, (Criterion C) avoidance, and (Criterion D) hyperarousal. Identifying the specific Criterion A1 event can be akin to that of chronic captivity situations, which lack a single identifiable traumatic stressor. Moreover, because of the chronicity of the autism-related exposure, ongoing intrusion occurs. This same ongoing exposure makes literal avoidance all but impossible, encouraging numbing as a psychological avoidance strategy. For example, one parent of a child with autism stated,

> [in an effort to stop him running out into the road] I have lately taken to making him read any article in the newspaper about pedestrians, especially children, being killed by cars. What frightens me the most is that these near-misses happen so frequently, I'm almost becoming accustomed and numb to them. This last incident had a sense of unreality. The horror didn't actually reach me this time as it has in the past, at least not consciously. The driver and the other mom seemed far more shaken up than me. I was thinking of that idea of flight, fright, or freeze–but it's a freeze that won't seem to thaw.

Hyperarousal symptoms are fed by the constant exposure to highly affectively-charged environment brought about by living with a person who is constantly on the move, potentially engaging in high-risk behaviors, and who may emit frightening or nerve-wracking sounds in their attempt to communicate. The constant vigilance to protect ones' child, one's family, and one's partner as well as one's self can leave parents irritable and on edge indefinitely. These symptoms may cause clinically significant problems in daily social and occupational functioning, both from the perspective of PTSD and other physical and mental/behavioral health perspectives.

Deepening the suffering of these families is the fact that it is difficult to construct a reasonable reality and interpret the experiences with which they are confronted (McCann & Pearlman, 1990). As a result of the person with autism's impaired social awareness, they may show no remorse, no reciprocation of appreciation, or no normally expected signs of love. This leaves families wondering if their children are indeed happy, if they care about or love their families, and, always, if "we are doing the right thing."

Yet another cause of stress to the family is the lack of general awareness about the disorder on the part of the general public. The child with autism has no physical characteristics to indicate that there is a disability. When the family attempts to go out in public, they may be shamed or embarrassed if the autistic child enacts bizarre behaviors. People may assign blame to the child's parents for these unusual behaviors. As is common with stigma, feelings of being judged and rejected may cause parents to isolate themselves (Miller & Sammons, 1999), further reducing their coping resources.

Added to this humiliation is the vestige of shame caused by the previously accepted, but misguided, medical hypothesis that cold or abusive parenting caused autism (Rimland, 1984). In the past and occasionally still, doctors remove the child from the care of the family and place the child in an institution, suggesting that the parents seek professional help for their own problems. Families who are otherwise confident that they have not abused their children wonder, "Did I let him cry too long in his crib? Should I have held him more as an infant? Did I give him enough time and love?" Because there are no clear answers to what causes autism, parents may speculate that they caused the autism.

Today, it is an ongoing challenge for the members of a family with an autistic child to adjust to the reality of their situation and find fulfillment together (Siegel, 1996). The cost of therapy and education for an autistic child is enormous. In most places, there is no day care or after-school care for the child with autism. Finding a babysitter who can deal with the disruptive and dangerous behaviors is extremely difficult. The problem of constant care for the child may prevent parents from working or spending time together. Given the stress and the financial drain on the family, the parents are at high risk for marital conflict as well as divorce (Seligman & Darling, 1997).

GROWING INCIDENCE AND AWARENESS

In the last decade, there has been an explosion in the number of new cases of autism-related disorders. The Autism Society of America (ASA) estimates between 500,000 and 1.5 million people in the United States alone have a disorder on the autism spectrum (ASA, 2002). Whereas the incidence was estimated at 1 in 5,000 births in the 1970s (Gerlai, 2004), now some studies are referencing up to 1 in 149 births (Centers for Disease Control and Prevention, 2000). Researchers and families are struggling to discern if this is truly an epidemic or due to better diagnosis.

A recent study reported by the *Journal of the American Medical Association* (Yeargin-Allsopp, Rice, Karapurkar, Doernberg, Boyle, & Murphy, 2003) reported the prevalence of autism among children aged 3 to 10 years in the 5 counties of metropolitan Atlanta, Georgia, in 1996. Cases were identified through screening and abstracting records from multiple medical and educational sources, with case status determined by expert review. A total of 987 children displayed behaviors consistent with autistic disorder, pervasive developmental disorder–not otherwise specified, or Asperger's syndrome. The prevalence for autism was 3.4 per 1000. Overall, the prevalence was comparable for black and white children, and 68 percent of children tested ($n = 880$) showed some type of cognitive impairment. The rate of autism found in this study was higher than the rates reported during the 1980s and early 1990s. While some of the increase can be explained by widened definitions of the disorder, Yeargin-Allsopp and colleagues claim that the cause for the increase is unknown. This increase is consistent with other recent studies, such as done by the M.I.N.D. Institute at the UC Davis Health System in California. M.I.N.D. reported a 273% increase in autism cases between 1987 and 1998 (Byrd, 1999), and also concluded that broadening the diagnostic criteria and other proposed factors do not account for this increase.

USING TECHNOLOGY TO REDUCE RISK FACTORS AND INCREASE PROTECTIVE FACTORS FOR CHILDREN AND THEIR FAMILY MEMBERS

The rising incidence of autism with concomitant limited professional resources has led to more consideration for using technology to link families and professionals, and to implement strategies to improve the outcomes for individuals with autism and their families. These are reviewed in context of the unique health, education, and the current family/professional support issues facing those dealing with autism.

Healthcare

Various challenges in delivering healthcare may exacerbate the distress of living with autism. For example, access to appointments with the relatively few professionals experienced in dealing with autism is limited and families may wait for weeks or months for an appointment. Even if they are fortunate enough to get appointments immediately, families far from major medical centers must often travel great distances to gain access to the relatively few autism experts. Once there, the individual with autism may not demonstrate the target behavior or, at the other extreme, cannot adapt to the clinical environment, thus preventing a useful examination. Families often struggle to convey to neurologists, psychologists, and psychiatrists behaviors or side effects of medication in order to get appropriate and accurate intervention earlier, or they may be too distressed to present well their family member's medical history.

Given a history of medical misunderstanding of the disease and many parents' feelings of guilt, a mistrust of the medical community may develop. The relationship becomes even more tenuous when a health care professional has little understanding of autism and can provide no relief to either the child or the family. The family is confronted again with the feeling that they are alone with no help. This alienation can continue for months and years until they locate specialists with the expertise they need for their child, and until they connect with and find support in other families who are coping with similar issues. As Naseef (2001) notes, parents' relationships with professionals are born of necessity and desperation during a time of grief and are therefore rife with opportunities for misunderstanding and conflict. No one wants to spend countless hours having his or her child diagnosed and treated in the offices, clinics, hospitals, and special schools by doctors, therapists, psychologists, teachers, and social workers. Families simply want someone to fix their child, fulfill their dreams, and take their pain away.

One family's recounting of their son's health issues is typical of the problems encountered by families:

After Jesse's first 15 months, we started to sense differences in his development, as compared with our two older children. We spent the following year nervously and repeatedly visiting our pediatrician to seek reasons for Jesse's gradual loss of language, peculiar and challenging behaviors, crying tantrums, and periods of unresponsiveness. We also went beyond the pediatrician's guidance and had Jesse's hearing tested and an EEG done.

When his preschool handicapped class psychologist finally threw out the possibility of autism, a neurologist fit us in for a formal evaluation (still took us two months) and confirmed a diagnosis of autism within five minutes of looking at Jesse. We struggled through many doctor visits to rule out sore throats, earaches, and other medical ailments that Jesse was not able to communicate. We made these visits as a last resort, because we dreaded Jesse's intermittent screaming outbursts in a full waiting room (I still do not know what it is about this environment that precipitates these outbursts).

Seven years later, we have now been to four different health professionals for autism and have re-told Jesse's history of care (my husband and I still disagree about what really worked and what did not, including such treatments as auditory training and dietary intervention). We do not know whom to go to next, and disagree about whether Jesse should be put on medication to treat his increasingly frequent self-injuring rages. We've already spent roughly $20,000 in self-funded medical expenses. (TalkAutism, 2003)

How Telehealth Can Help

Telehealth is the use of electronic information and telecommunications technologies to support long-distance clinical health care, patient and professional health-related education, public health, and health administration. Use of telehealth has expanded rapidly since the 1990s and is becoming an effective means for increasing access to healthcare (Office for the Advancement of Telehealth [OAT], 2003). *Real-time* (synchronous) telehealth or telemedicine includes videoconferencing between provider and patient, or consultations between providers. *Store-and-forward* (asynchronous) telehealth or telemedicine involves capturing medical information electronically, and forwarding this to a health professional for review (Stamm, 1998). Care must be taken to protect patient confidentiality, but there are multiple technology options to assure the security of the transmitted data.

Because it is difficult to accurately sample usual behavior during an office visit, store and forward telemedicine improve a provider's understanding of the person's behavior and subsequently their treatment plan. Figure 1 demonstrates a simple strategy of capturing a behavioral sample to share with a health provider. The strategy is as follows: (a) caretakers videotape an episode of concern or interest (the episode is automatically time-stamped); (b) the video is mailed conventionally or is electronically transferred to the appropriate health professional; (c) the health professional then reviews the video, (d) responds via

FIGURE 1. Flow Diagram for Using Telemedicine with Autism

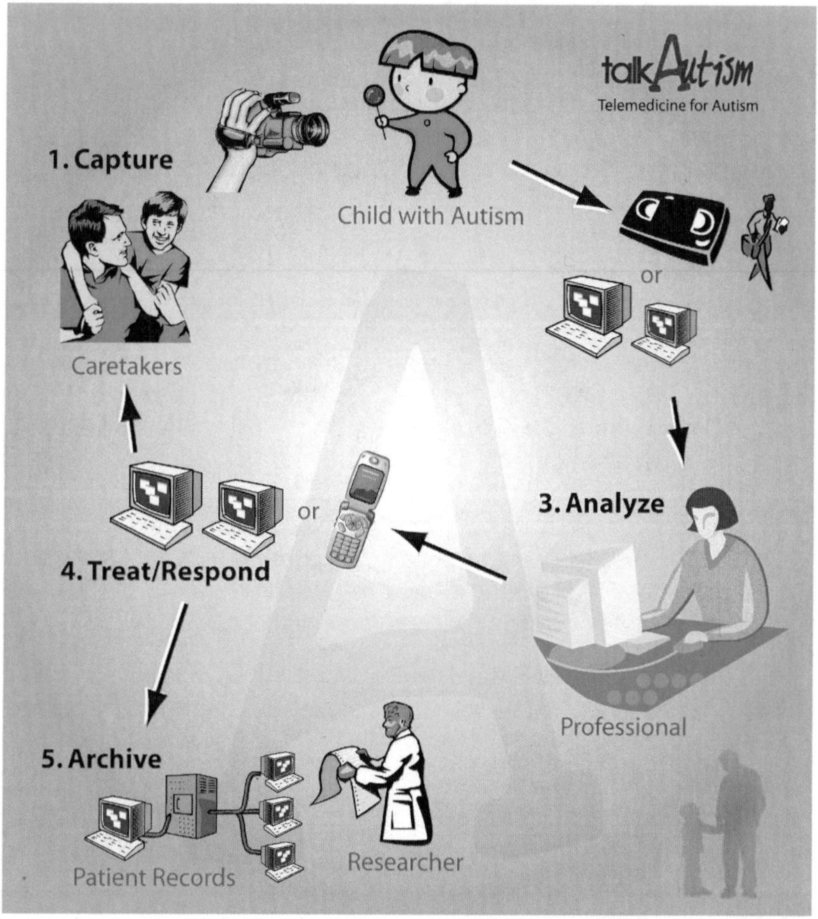

phone, letter, or e-mail, and (e) archives the episode for future reference and research (Princeton Autism Technology [PAT], 2003).

This simple technology can lessen the distress of living with autism by giving families a more effective method for communicating unique health, behavioral, and educational issues such as episodes of self-injury, seizures, tantrums, or aggression. At least one study found this type of patient-provider communication reduced overall stress and saved time and money (Grady, 2002). Additionally, with video-imaging modalities, health professionals have a better understanding of what is happening to children in their own natural environments at the time of the episode, while simultaneously creating a more extensive medical record for diagnosis, follow-up to prescribing of medication, family counseling, and their own continuing medical education.

An electronic medical record makes it easier to link information that may be missed in a paper record (see Table 1). For example, videos showing behaviors, lab reports showing physiology, neuroimaging showing anatomy, and EKG readings showing neurology all on one patient record offer a more complete picture of the patient's condition, and should facilitate current clinical reference or when multiple health professionals will be involved over a patient's life. In addition, aggregating across patient records can offer researchers opportunities for identifying patterns across patients leading to clues about the disorder.

Several 'autism' programs currently use various forms of this telemedicine to assist families. For example, the National Rehabilitation Hospital (Washington, DC) uses videophones to provide an ongoing presence in the homes of their patients, while the University of Arizona has made autism diagnoses via interactive video for patients in families living in rural areas. Eden Institute (Princeton, NJ), a school for children with autism, has used videoconferencing to communicate with a psychiatrist 300 miles away for diagnoses and for monitoring students' medications (Eden Institute Outreach Director, personal communication, June 3,

TABLE 1. A Note About the Electronic Medical Record

An electronic medical record (EMR) is a repository of clinically pertinent data that may be accessed and searched with relative ease. In digital form, medical records can be automatically scanned for everything from potential drug interactions to lab reports to gaps in clinical data (Bergeron, 1998). So much of the current treatment of children with autism relies on parents' ability to convey a helpful history of their children's health and behavior problems. Electronic medical records may help correlate complex and extensive medical histories effectively. These can be stored at one doctor's office, at home, or on a secure Web server, providing multiple health professionals access to one patient's unique medical history.

2003). Finally, in various clinics, health professionals have used video-tapes sent in from families of patients to effectively counsel the families on treatment options. In some cases, insurance companies have reimbursed these encounters (Weitzen, 2003).

Specialists from various disciplines, including those in neurology, psychiatry, psychology, social work, counseling, speech and language, occupational therapy, and physical therapy can utilize telehealth. As families are secure in their relationships with the professionals who are their partners and guides in their child's development, they can begin to regain a sense of hope about their family's future, thus mediating some families' tendencies toward PTSD.

Education

Early intervention and a highly structured education program are regarded currently as the best treatments for children with autism, offering the best chance for normal schooling and a more typical life. One-on-one specialized therapy sessions (frequently referred to as applied behavior analysis [ABA], which uses simple tasks to shape the child's behavior by rewarding target behaviors with praise, food, or other tangible rewards) for up to 40 hours per week have allowed over 50% of the children researched to be integrated into regular classrooms and community activities (Lovass, 1987). Maintaining this highly structured therapy is difficult due to financial and treatment constraints that range from interfamilial to community based issues. Families look to professionals to guide them and help their child. However, because of budgetary problems or philosophical differences, parents and school districts can find themselves in conflict about what type or scope of special education is appropriate for the child. This conflict can set up the family and school district as adversaries almost from initial diagnosis. The following anecdote from a parent on TalkAutism (2003) message board demonstrates this:

> When we brought little Alex (5 years old), our nonverbal child with autism, to his first ever "special ed" class, we were unsettled by the fact that he was in a class that did not specialize in autism. After a series of drawn-out meetings with the over-worked child-study team that spanned months, we inquired why the school would not abide the education regimen of 40 hours per week of intensive therapy cited in Dr. Lovass' study. "We're doing everything we can," said the well-meaning learning consultant. We hear rumors about the

> school is already over-budget in special ed due to the influx of students with autism. (TalkAutism, 2003)

With the increasing incidence of autism, school districts are trying to stay ahead of the exploding numbers of cases, increasing the pressure on school districts' special services programs. However, many school districts fall short of both parent and teacher expectations when it comes to actual management of the classroom and adhering to the students' Individual Educational Plans (IEPs) (Mayerson, 2003). Some dedicated private schools provide an out-of-district option, but due to a growing trend toward community integration and the Individuals with Disabilities Education Act (IDEA) requirement that students be taught in the *least restrictive environment* (LRE), more school districts are attempting to establish their own.

Public school districts typically look outside their district to "consultation models" for guidance in establishing their programs. A typical consultation model begins by training staff about autism and the educational philosophy that will be utilized; this training is followed up with weekly or monthly visits to provide feedback and ongoing training. Among the many challenges inherent in this model are the ongoing supervision needs of staff, the occurrence of unique episodes requiring immediate consultant guidance, data collection to gauge progress, the breadth of educational autism-related techniques needed by teachers, and the demands of supplemental home programs to support families. In addition, staff turnover is a chronic problem for school districts and has a particularly negative effect when teachers with specialized skills leave.

What Videoconferencing Can Do

Videoconferencing is two-way electronic communications system that permits two or more persons in different locations to see and hear each other. Attached computers or video recording devices can be used to archive encounters for later referencing. The quality of videoconferencing is related to the available bandwidth and can range from stand-alone units that offer broadcast quality to attachments on personal computers or low-cost videophones that use the same wiring that traditional phones do (see Table 2).

Several autism programs currently use various forms of this telehealth technology to support schools working with children with autism and their families. For example, Youth Consultation Services (YCS; Montclair, NJ) is using videophones successfully to connect its relatively few experts in highly specialized areas with "green" school districts in different parts of the country, providing "hands on" guidance while reducing travel. YCS records and archives exercises to facilitate identification of where improvements are occurring. With confidentiality issues addressed, it uses the recordings for ongoing training of the frontline professionals. A second example is the company Advoserv out of Bear (Delaware), which uses interactive videoconference to connect experienced behavioral consultants who can supervise paraprofessionals or work directly with young adults with autism in work programs to assist them with work skills remotely (Baker, 2003).

Some groups are piloting studies in which education professionals are testing videoconferencing to augment families' access to therapists (PAT, 2003). By directly connecting schools and homes through videoconferencing and information technology, families may have increased and more efficient access to professional resources, thereby helping to reduce the distress families experience (see Table 3).

TABLE 2. A Note About Video Capture

Videotaping students' progress has already been a common tool used because of the usefulness to observe movement and sounds to note a student's baseline and progress. With the advent of digital capturing devices and "video stream," video capture is easier to facilitate, and now allows instantaneous means to forward via the Internet to specialists who may not be present. Archiving these video clips in a digital database for reference should provide new data mining opportunities for research.

TALBE 3. A Note About Teletheraphy

We are not aware of any trials that investigate videoconferencing as an augmentation of "one-on-one" intensive therapy between therapist and student described and recommended by Lovass and others. There are currently numerous users of videoconferencing (businesspeople, university students, and now even prisoners), and we believe that many students with autism have an innate capability for interacting with this modality effectively. Would this technology thus boost the results from today's intensive one-on-one therapy?

To suggest one application, these videoconference systems could also allow the therapist to provide customized *multimedia awards* on the students' monitors to keep them interested and motivated. If this application of videoconferencing works, the relatively few expert therapists in the field could better regulate the time they spend with each child, and staff turnover might be reduced if professionals could work from their own home to work with children who may be miles away. Some psychiatrists have observed that prisoners become more responsive in a teletherapy environment. We recommend that trials using videoconferencing to deliver *teletherapy* should be launched in the autism arena as well.

What Computer Technology Can Do

Computer technology includes both computer hardware (from personal computers to palm-sized hand-held devices) and software. Computer technology is used more and more to augment the education of people with autism.

There is a perception that people with autism are adept with computer technology, such as that alluded to in articles like *Wired Magazine*'s "The Geek Syndrome" (Silberman, 2001).

> Many students with autism are highly interested and motivated by computers. Therefore, computers should be infused into the child's daily curriculum, not used solely for reward or recreational purposes. Computer assisted learning can focus on numerous academic areas as well as provide an appropriate independent leisure time activity for people with autism. Computers are motivating to children with autism, due to their predictability and consistency, compared to the unpredictable nature of human responses (Hileman, 1996). The computer does not send confusing social messages. The computer places the child in control, allowing for the child to become an independent learner. (Stokes, 2001)

A growing number of software companies have created programs that build on techniques for teaching children with autism (see Table 4).

An increasingly important use of existing computer technology for the future could be to provide automated tabulation functions on computers and hand-held personal computing devices (PDAs) to record a child's specific activities. Such technology can save time and improve

TABLE 4. Computer Technology Examples (PAT, 2003)

- Software programs to re-create a teacher's one-on-one exercises, even inserting virtual props and "mimicking the teacher's voice," if desired (e.g., www.learninghelper.com).
- Software programs to help children with autism make gains in the language and listening skills necessary for reading (e.g., www.fastforword.com).
- Assistive technology devices include "speaking" touch pad laptop computer devices to facilitate the communication of people with autism who are nonverbal (e.g., www.dynavoxsys. com).
- Web-based programs that provide an online virtual reality environment that allows children with autism to practice important skills such as evacuating a burning house (e.g., www.do2learn.org).

observation, data assimilation, and reporting, all of which can improve the child's learning and school-family interactions. Data can be centralized, allowing for timely sharing of information and easing the stress on parents, who no longer have to go through several other people to keep up with their children's progress, as well as assist teachers with record keeping and communication sharing.

Supporting Families and Professionals

Those working with a person with autism, whether they are family or professionals, endure many conditions that affect their ability to cope with the aspects of autism. Beyond coordinating the regimens of healthcare and special education described earlier, family members may feel a continuing responsibility to search for something else that may help, something that perhaps may not yet have surfaced because of the poor communication in the autism community and the lack of efficacy research. Compounding their anguish is the need to be close to home to care for the child with autism. Together, uncertainty and isolation intensify the distress besetting these families. Professionals also struggle to keep up with the ever-changing medical, legal, and educational aspects of autism. Recent breakthroughs in diagnosis and treatment, more state-of-the-science meetings, and even full education programs are reason for hope, yet word of these developments is reaching relatively few who can attend conferences that are often filled to capacity.

Pediatricians are on the "frontline" in diagnosing people with autism accurately and many more health practitioners will subsequently treat these patients' "family medicine" needs. However, health professionals are without the in-depth and up-to-date information and training to do so. Up to six million special education workforces in 15,000 school districts in the United States need continuing education to implement evidence based education protocols.

In general, autism organizations supporting families and health and education professionals with information and training have been mostly volunteer, have been poorly funded, and have struggled to leverage technology to improve their access to their constituents. There is a need for better communication to enable professionals to share expertise and technologies with education professionals and paraprofessionals, and with the families and relatives in the autism lay community. As one parent recalls:

I remember the 100-mile drive home from the last doctor visit to our Nebraska farmhouse, openly crying about my son's diagnosis of "autism." I didn't believe the neurologist's assessment of "there's not much you can do about it," and vowed during that drive to research the treatments that would "cure my son." Searching the Internet, I was at first encouraged to see 990,000 responses to "autism" in one of the search engines, but I soon felt disheartened when much of the prevalent available support material was itself dated, white washed, and comparable in perspective to the professional assessment I received. I saw there were several conferences, but these were months away and in cities on the east or west coast. (TalkAutism, 2003)

What Distance Education Can Do

The future of education in our society will most certainly bear witness to the increased use of technology for teaching and learning at all levels. Distance education is defined as a formal educational process in which the majority of the instruction occurs when student and instructor are not in the same place. Instruction may be synchronous or asynchronous. Distance education may employ correspondence study, or audio, video, or computer technologies. Applications of this technology range from videoconferencing that features live presentations to text-based courses accessed through mail or the Internet, and many variations in between. Accreditation and e-commerce are also facilitated. Its widescale acceptance is expected to increase at a rate of 40% annually for the foreseeable future (Gallagher, 2002).

Distance education provides an effective way of disseminating new findings, as well as already established programs and courses, and of reinforcing the curriculum taught at conferences and seminars. With its unique challenges, the autism "community" is ideal to benefit from this technology. Autism-specific distance education examples already in use are listed in Table 5.

Distance learning applications can lessen the distress of living with autism by providing information to isolated families, especially those living in rural or underserved communities. Parents and professionals alike can learn state-of-the-art treatment techniques, allowing them to feel that they are doing all that is possible for people with autism in their care.

TABLE 5. Distance Education Examples Already in Use Related to Autism

- Providing online learning environments that promote educational tools and programs for children and adults with special learning needs, including free teacher and parent materials, computer-based instruction (safety games, learning games, language games) (e.g., www.do2learn.org).
- Specialty Chats that allow free access to experts online for parents and professionals thru an online chat room environment, with archive abilities to help those not able to attend (e.g., www.talkautism.org, www.reedmartin.com).
- Online lectures provided via video-streaming or text-based courses via the Internet that enable experts to teach professionals and families about autism (e.g., www.dougflutiejrfoundation.org, www.autismtoday.com, www.talkautism.org, and www.poac.net).
- Use of webcasting and videoconference to more broadly disseminate conference proceedings used by several organizations.

What Information Technology Can Do

Information technology refers to the collection of products and services that turn data into useful, meaningful, accessible information (Information Technology Association of America [ITAA], 2003). Our use of this term encompasses related internet technologies that facilitate families' access to knowledge, information, and assistance. Information technology can increase communication, speed research, and coalesce different groups' efforts to support families and advocate for changes in the caliber of care and services. There continues to be a growth in networks, primarily using the Internet, that enable families to console each other, advocate for services and research, and access expert opinion and resources.

Applications of information technology to autism are varied. For example, there are interactive Websites that allow members of a child's intervention team to access IEPs, progress reports, and all the other data that has been collected. The platforms can house videos of best-practice procedures, document libraries containing forms and templates to facilitate executing individual education plans (e.g., www.verbalbehaviornet work.com). In addition, there are more than 500 online listservs, message boards, archiving databases, and Internet newsletters serving the autism community (TalkAutism, 2003).

By (a) uniting the numerous small advocacy groups that have been isolated historically, (b) connecting families online who can learn from others with similar challenges, or (c) disseminating latest findings to professionals and families, distance education and information technology can help the community more effectively advocate and obtain significant support.

CONCLUSION

The stress experienced by family members who deal with autism is unique and overwhelming at times, and may put them at risk for PTSD and/or its sub-syndromal variants. The rising incidence of autism and growing public awareness about the disorder have prompted an ever more audible demand for appropriate services, support, and research. Many of the increased services and supports are available or can soon be using technology. Technology is not a magic wand that will make autism go away, but it can make a significant difference in the lives of people with autism, their families, and their social and professional support system by quickly and efficiently marshaling medical consultation, behavioral interventions, and other services and supports. Research can be fostered and disseminated. Teachers and therapists can benefit from state-of-the-art training and collaboration. The applications described function as tools to lessen the stress on families and, simultaneously, as catalysts to research, prevention, and intervention.

NOTE

1. While we use the term *family member*, we recognize that other caregivers, professional and volunteer, may be similarly affected as a result of their closeness with the person with autism.

REFERENCES

Akshoomoff, N. (2000). Neurological underpinnings of autism. In A. Wetherby & B. Prizant (Eds.), *Autism spectrum disorders: A transactional development perspective* (pp. 167-192). Baltimore: Paul Brookes Publishing.

American Psychiatric Association. (2000). *Diagnostic and statistical manual of mental disorders* (4th ed., text rev.). Washington, DC: Author.

Antonovsky, A. (1979). *Health, stress, and coping: New perspectives on mental and physical well-being.* San-Francisco: Jossey-Bass.

Antonovsky, A. (1987). *Unraveling the mystery of health: How people manage stress and stay well.* San Francisco: Jossey-Bass.

Autism Society of America. (2002). *ASA President's testimony to Congress.* Retrieved June 22, 2003 from, www.autism-society.org

Baker, L., Thwing, G., Shea, T., McGimsey, J., & Favell, J. (2003). *Examining the efficacy of delivering professional services in human service settings through the use of interactive video.* Report to Health to Human Services, Administration on Children and Families. On File at C Now (Mt. Dora, FL).

Bergeron, B. P. (1998, July). Can electronic medical records really achieve information sharing? *Postgraduate Medicine Online, 104*(7). Available from, http://www.postgradmed.com/issues/1998/07_98/dd_jul98.htm

Bristol, M. M. (1984). Family resources and successful adaptation to autistic children. In E. Schopler & G. B. Meisbov (Eds.), *The effects of autism on the family* (pp. 289-310). New York: Plenum.

Byrd, R. (1999). *Changes in the population of persons with autism or pervasive developmental disorders in California's Development Services System: 1987 to 1998. Report to the Legislature.* Retrieved June 15, 2003 from, http://www.dds.ca.gov/Autism/pdf/Autism_Report_1999.PDF

Centers for Disease Control and Prevention. (2000). *Prevalence of autism in Brick Township, New Jersey, 1998 Community Report.* Retrieved June 16, 2003 from, http://www.cdc.gov/ncbddd/dd/report.htm

Durand, V. D. (1998). *Sleep better: A guide to improving sleep for children with special needs.* Baltimore: Paul Brookes Publishing.

Gallagher, S. (2002) *Distance learning at the tipping point, September,* Eduventures. Retrieved May 5, 2004 from, http://www.eduventures.com/pdf/distance.pdf

Gerlai, R., & Gerlai, J. (2004). Autism: A target of pharmacotherapies? *Drug Discovery Today, 9*(8), 366-372.

Grady, B. J. (2002). A comparative cost analysis of an integrated military telemental health-care service. *Telemedicine Journal and e-Health, 8*(3), 293-300.

Greenspan, S., & Weider, S. (1999). *The child with special needs: Encouraging intellectual and emotional growth.* Reading, MA: Addison Wesley

Herman, J. (1992). *Trauma and recovery: The aftermath of violence–from domestic abuse to political terror.* New York: Basic Books.

Hileman, C. (1996, July). *Computer technology with autistic children.* Paper presented at the annual Autism Society of America National Conference, Milwaukee, WI.

Information Technology Association of America. (2003). *About ITAA.* Retrieved June 14, 2003 from, www.itaa.org

Janoff-Bulman, R. (1992). *Shattered assumptions: Towards a new psychology of trauma.* New York: Free Press.

Lovass, O. I. (1987). Behavioral treatment and normal educational and intellectual functioning in young autistic children. *Journal of Consulting and Clinical Psychology, 55,* 3-9.

Mayerson, G. S. (2003). How to try an autism case. *New Jersey Lawyer: Special Education Law Issue,* 28-34.

McCann, L., & Pearlman, L. A. (1990). *Psychological trauma and the adult survivor: Theory, therapy, and transformation.* New York: Brunner-Routledge.

Miller, N., & Sammons, C. (1999). *Everybody's different: Understanding and changing our reactions to disabilities.* Baltimore, MD: Paul Brookes Publishing.

Naseef, R. (2001) *Special children, challenged parents: The struggles and rewards of raising a child with a disability.* Baltimore, MD: Paul Brookes Publishing.

Newman, E., Christopher, S. R., & Berry, J. O. (2000). Developmental disabilities, trauma exposure, and post-traumatic stress disorder. *Trauma, Violence, and Abuse: A Review Journal 1,* 154-170.

Office for the Advancement of Telehealth. (2003). *Office for the Advancement of Telehealth–Welcome Page.* Retrieved 21 July 2003, from http://telehealth. hrsa.gov/welcome.htm

Princeton Autism Technology. (2003). *PAT's ExpertFind resource directory.* Retrieved June 15, 2003 from, www.autismtechnology.org.

Rimland, B. (1984). *Infantile autism.* New York: Irvington Publishing.

Seligman, S., & Darling, R. B. (1997). *Ordinary families, special children: A systems approach to childhood disability.* New York: Guilford Press.

Siegel, B. (1996). *The world of the autistic child: Understanding and treating autistic spectrum disorders.* New York: Oxford University Press.

Silberman, S. (2001). The geek syndrome. *Wired Magazine, 9*(12). Available from, http://www.wired.com/wired/archive/9.12/aspergers_pr.html

Stamm, B. H. (1998). Clinical applications of telehealth in mental health care. *Professional Psychology: Research and Practice, 29*(6), 536-542.

Stamm, B. H. (1999a). Empirical perspectives on contextualizing death and trauma. In C. R. Figley (Ed.), *Traumatology of grieving* (pp. 23-36). Philadelphia: Brunner/Mazel.

Stamm, B. H. (1999b). Theoretical perspectives on contextualizing death and trauma. In C. R. Figley (Ed.), *Traumatology of grieving* (pp. 3-21). Philadelphia: Brunner/Mazel.

Stern, D. M., & Bruschweiler-Stern, N. (1998). *The birth of a mother: How the motherhood experience changes you forever.* New York: Basic Books.

Stokes, S. (2001). *Assistive technology for children with autism.* Report published for Wisconsin Department of Public Instruction. Retrieved June 15, 2003 from, http://www.cesa7.k12.wi.us/sped/autism/assist/asst10.htm

TalkAutism. (2003). A coalition-based communication service shared by several autism organizations to facilitate online communication and access to resources. Message board excerpts retrieved June 9-15, 2003 from, www.talkautism.org/DA.asp

van der Kolk, B. A., McFarlane, A. C., & Weisaeth, L. (Eds.) (1996). *Traumatic stress: The effects of overwhelming experience on mind, body, and society.* New York: Guilford.

Weitzen, G. (2003, March 15). *Guest speaker on TalkAutism. Virtual speaker specialty chat: Finding resources locally.* Retrieved June 14, 2003 from, www.talkautism. org/VS.asp

Yeargin-Allsopp, M., Rice, C., Karapurkar, T., Doernberg, N., Boyle, C., & Murphy, C. (2003). Prevalence of autism in a US metropolitan area. *Journal of the American Medical Association, 289,* 49-55.

Index

Action stage, PTSD model, 12
Acupressure points, emotional freedom
    technique, 126,135
Acute stress disorder (ASD)
    PTSD, 35,94
    thought field therapy, 104
Addiction, complex PTSD, 33
Adjustment disorder, 94
Aggression, complex PTSD, 33
Aging, attention deficit, 15
Agoraphobia
    complex PTSD, 47
    diagnosis, 89,95
Alarcon, R. D., xv,199
Alcohol abuse model, 10
American Medical Association
    (AMA), 93
American Psychiatric Association, 2,
    93
American Psychological Association,
    61
Anatomy of an Illness (Cousins), 172
Angelou, M., 176
Anger management, PTSD, 11
Anhedonia, 175
Anxiety
    complex PTSD, 34
    humor, 173
    managing, 171
Anxiety disorders
    diagnosis, 89,95
    muscle testing, 111
    PTSD, 94
    thought field therapy, 127
Applied behavior analysis (ABA), 233
Arousal reduction, complex PTSD, 40
Art therapy
    expression, 187
    flexibility, 191

    grandmother group, 191
    interpreter role, 185
    men's groups, 188
    PTSD, 187
    target groups, 184
    terrorist attacks, 73
    trauma survivors, 183
    war refugees, 5,183
Association for Thought Field
    Therapy, 120
Association of Traumatic Stress
    Specialists, 73,118
Autism
    Atlanta, 228
    California, 225
    case history, 230
    children, 222,228
    computer technology, 236
    consultation models, 234
    defining, 223
    diagnosis, 223
    distance education, 238
    education programs, 233
    electronic medical record, 232
    family at risk, 224-227
    healthcare, 229
    incidence, 222,228
    information technology, 239
    misconceptions, 227
    neurological damage, 222
    new techniques, 221,228
    pediatricians, 239
    PTSD, 222
    protective factors, 228
    public awareness, 227
    risk factors, 228
    software programs, 236
    stress factor, 222
    support groups, 237

precise and specific, 112
PTSD patients, 114
school shootings, 105
self-care, 118
sexual assault, 107
SUDS, 115
trauma protocol, 116,122
traumatic stress, 103,116
Web sites, 120
Trauma
anthropologist view, 1
art therapy, 183
Bosnian refugees, 186
debriefing interventions, 57,67
defining, 154,225
early responses, 69
emotional freedom technique, 125
humor of survivors, 169
information guidelines, 69-74
interpreter role, 185
perception, 2
post-event activities, 77
psychotherapy, 2
repression, 155
resilience and coping, 75
safety and routine, 68
school response, 57,67
techniques, 3-6
Traumatic incident reduction (TIR)
affect intensity, 162
applications, 165
awareness threshold, 158
case study, 165
detail and steps, 157-161
earlier incidents, 163
energy drain, 155
exposure technique, 151
facilitator role, 164
limitations, 165
person-centered, 151
protocol, 158
PTSD, 151,156,165
research, 165
root sequence, 156
safe environment, 164

session pattern, 161
when and where, 159

University of Arizona, 232
University of California (Davis), 228

Veterans
attention deficit, 15
case studies, 212-216
humor, 170
patient selection, 204
PTSD, 199,203
virtual reality exposure, 199,202
Veterans Administration Medical
Centers (VAMC)
Atlanta, 200,206,217
New Orleans, 23
PTSD treatment, 9,23,200,206
virtual reality exposure, 206,217
Video conferencing, autism, 235
Vietnam veterans
case studies, 212-216
humor, 170
PTSD, 200,203
Virtual reality exposure (VRE)
advantages, 202
body memories, 214
case studies, 212-216
head-mounted display, 202
lifestyle changes, 215
measures and procedures, 205-209
method and results, 204-212
outcome measures, 211
patient selection, 204
phobias, 216
PTSD veterans, 199,202
rationale, 203
terrorist attack, 217
treatment schedule, 207
typical session, 209

BOOK ORDER FORM!

Order a copy of this book with this form or online at:
http://www.HaworthPress.com/store/product.asp?sku=5544

Trauma Treatment Techniques
Innovative Trends

_____ in softbound at $39.95 ISBN-13: 978-0-7890-2844-0 / ISBN-10: 0-7890-2844-1.
_____ in hardbound at $59.95 ISBN-13: 978-0-7890-2843-3 / ISBN-10: 0-7890-2843-3.

COST OF BOOKS _____

POSTAGE & HANDLING _____
US: $4.00 for first book & $1.50
for each additional book
Outside US: $5.00 for first book
& $2.00 for each additional book.

SUBTOTAL _____
In Canada: add 7% GST. _____

STATE TAX _____
CA, IL, IN, MN, NJ, NY, OH, PA & SD residents
please add appropriate local sales tax.

FINAL TOTAL _____
If paying in Canadian funds, convert
using the current exchange rate,
UNESCO coupons welcome.

❑**BILL ME LATER:**
Bill-me option is good on US/Canada/
Mexico orders only; not good to jobbers,
wholesalers, or subscription agencies.

❑ **Signature** _____

❑ **Payment Enclosed: $** _____

❑ **PLEASE CHARGE TO MY CREDIT CARD:**

❑Visa ❑MasterCard ❑AmEx ❑Discover
❑Diner's Club ❑Eurocard ❑JCB

Account # _____

Exp Date _____

Signature _____

(Prices in US dollars and subject to change without notice.)

PLEASE PRINT ALL INFORMATION OR ATTACH YOUR BUSINESS CARD

Name	
Address	
City	State/Province	Zip/Postal Code
Country	
Tel	Fax
E-Mail	

May we use your e-mail address for confirmations and other types of information? ❑Yes ❑No We appreciate receiving
your e-mail address. Haworth would like to e-mail special discount offers to you, as a preferred customer.
We will never share, rent, or exchange your e-mail address. We regard such actions as an invasion of your privacy.

Order from your **local bookstore** or directly from
The Haworth Press, Inc. 10 Alice Street, Binghamton, New York 13904-1580 • USA
Call our toll-free number (1-800-429-6784) / Outside US/Canada: (607) 722-5857
Fax: 1-800-895-0582 / Outside US/Canada: (607) 771-0012
E-mail your order to us: orders@HaworthPress.com

For orders outside US and Canada, you may wish to order through your local
sales representative, distributor, or bookseller.
For information, see http://HaworthPress.com/distributors

(Discounts are available for individual orders in US and Canada only, not booksellers/distributors.)

The Haworth Press Inc.

Please photocopy this form for your personal use.
www.HaworthPress.com

BOF05